Praise for

"*Dr. Ed Park is on to something. A new way to age by turning back the clock!*"

— *Suzanne Somers, Best-selling author and wellness expert*

"*Dr. Park's book offers a clear and friendly account of the role of telomeres in causing age-related diseases and the enormous potential of telomerase to prevent and cure age-related diseases by reversing human aging at the genetic level. The tide is now racing in and Dr. Park is on top of the wave, leading the way for patients and clinicians worldwide.*"

— *Michael Fossel, MD, PhD.*
Author of "Reversing Human Aging" and
"Cells, Aging, and Human Disease"

"*Dr. Ed Park is one of America's leading physicians in personalized and preventative medicine – and one of the first to understand the clinical and critical importance of the biology of telomeres and telomere measurement as a biomarker for aging and health.*"

— *Stephen J. Matlin, CEO, Life Length*
(A leading company in telomere assessment)

"*In my view, Dr. Park has chosen the correct attitude for us to think about the process of aging...For example, he first asks, not if aging will be slowed, but 'When will aging become a thing of the past?' He then answers, 'Aging will soon become a choice rather than a curse.' Dr. Park's writing style and persuasive logic are a pleasure to read.*"

— *L. Stephen Coles, M.D., Ph.D.,*
UCLA's Gerontology Research Group

"If you know Ed Park the way I do you know that Ed Park has no trouble thinking outside the box. The result is Ed's explanations, logic, and organizational style in this work are spot on, entertaining and 100% unique- like Ed himself! If you are looking for a comforting rehash of what has been said and written before you won't find it here. Ed digs deep and pulls no punches. He basically says out loud what many of us think but are afraid to say. "Telomere Timebombs" is like no other book out there! Get it, read it and learn it, then use it to enlighten the world!"

— *Dave Woynarowski MD, Author of "The Immortality Edge"*

"If you want to know about living longer and healthier, Dr. Park is your man. If you want to know more about the origins of cancer and its treatment then Dr. Park is your man. His anecdotal studies are most impressive and speak to the effects of TA-65 on the action of telomeres and it seems that telomeres have been studied extensively allowing him to make statements about how long we can expect to live so if you care about a long life Dr. Park is your man."

— *Dr. Arthur Janov, Director, Primal Center, Santa Monica, CA*

TELOMERE TIMEBOMBS

Defusing the Terror of Aging

ED PARK, MD

Telomere Timebombs – Defusing the Terror of Aging
© 2013 Telomere Timebombs Publishing Inc. All rights reserved.
Ed Park, MD

No part of this book may be reproduced in any written, electronic, recording, or photocopying without written permission of the publisher or author.

Although every precaution has been taken to verify the accuracy of the information contained herein, the author and publisher assume no responsibility for any errors or omissions. No liability is assumed for damages that may result from the use of information contained within.

Telomerase activation medicine and telomere biology are rapidly-evolving areas so statements made herein may prove to be incomplete or inaccurate with the benefit of hindsight.

TA-65™ is a registered trademark of the T.A. Sciences Corporation of NY. The contents of this book do not necessarily represent the opinions of T.A. Sciences, The Geron Corporation, scientists mentioned within, nor anyone other than the author.

TA-65 is not FDA-approved for the prevention or treatment of any disease. Cases discussed are purely anecdotal and should not be construed to represent typical or expected effects of ingesting TA-65.

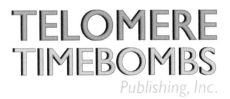

Books may be purchased by contacting the publisher at:
info@telomeretimebombs.com

Cover Design and Illustrations: Ed Park and Cecelia Snaith
Publisher: Telomere Timebombs Publishing, Inc. (Costa Mesa, CA)
ISBN: 978-0-9895837-0-1
10 9 8 7 6 5 4 3 2 1

1. Health 2. Medicine 3. Integrative Medicine 4. Telomere Biology

First Edition
Printed in the USA by Telomere Timebombs Publishing, Inc.

Dedication

First and foremost, I wish to dedicate this book to Cal Harley, former science officer of the Geron Corporation and Noel Patton, founder of T.A. Sciences, for making TA-65 available to mankind.

Secondly, this book is dedicated to my patients who had the courage, imagination, and faith to take this journey with me. You inspired me personally when times were challenging and continue to teach me about telomerase activation medicine every day.

I also dedicate this book to my friends and family for their love and support.

I also need to thank Susie Cyin for her good cheer and tireless support through these very interesting years.

And finally, I wish to thank whatever consciousness in the universe exists that has guided my actions, shown me such grace, and strengthened my faith despite my reluctance to call it by name.

Acknowledgements

How did this book come into existence? Well, our minds are always retelling our stories to make sense, assign meaning, and protect our egos from harm. But there are so many points of light in this constellation that it would be arbitrary and futile to list them all.

That said, I wish to thank the people who worked at the Geron Corporation, T.A. Sciences, PhysioAge, A4M, AMMG, Cathy Reinheimer and The Sun Valley Wellness Festival, the SmartLife Forum, Steve Coles and the GRG, and Suzanne Somers.

With regard to proof reading, I am grateful to Gentry Smith, Isabel Love, Jerine Watson, Claire McCurdy, and Gail Kay.

Special thanks to brilliant Cecelia Snaith for the inspired work she did realizing the cover design and illustrations.

Immeasurable gratitude goes out to the incomparable and sublime Gentry Smith for his support in designing and marketing the book, audio and ebook consulting, and website design and administration.

Finally thank you to anyone and everyone in my life's journey for bringing me closer to knowing myself, even if was not your intention and even if I didn't fully value your contribution at the time. I hope my presence in your life has made it a richer experience as well.

Contents

Table of Figures (by chapter and sequence)

INTRODUCTION

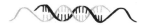

Thank you for picking up this book. It is an honor and a pleasure to share with you what I believe is the most important information that you need right now, to live your best and healthiest life.

The questions that you might be asking are:

- What is this book about and is it going to be interesting?
- Why should I care?
- How will this information help me?
- Is this going to be over my head, or will it be explained in a way that I can understand?
- Who is this Ed Park guy?
- When will aging become a thing of the past?

This book is about a revolutionary and simple way of thinking about health and aging. Your health and longevity are important. The concepts presented are so clear that a fifth grader will be able to explain them to you using simple analogies such as firecrackers, queen bees, and automobile repair.

My name is Ed Park and I am a medical doctor trained at Harvard and Columbia Universities and I am sharing what I've learned with you. This book is the result of years of experience and reflection while practicing what I call "telomerase activation medicine." As the book will explain, that entails using a plant-derived molecule to enhance the body's natural repair of its stem cells via an enzyme called telomerase.

My theories may be revolutionary, but I know without a doubt, they are true and self-evident. They are based entirely on scientific fact, experience, and thoughtful reflection.

So sit back, relax, and let me explain why I believe aging has already become a thing of the past. By the time you finish *Telomere Timebombs*, I know you will understand why telomerase activation ("TA" for short) is central to our healthy living. You will discover for yourself why the fantasy of staying alert, youthful, and vital is now within your grasp.

Before we start, I think I should prepare you for my style of writing in this book:

- I have chosen a very conversational tone, rather than a scientific or formal one. Yes, I know how to be serious and no, I don't want to write this particular book in that style.

- I use a lot of figurative language, like analogies and metaphors. We will switch but hopefully not mix metaphors quite frequently, so it may be a bit of a bumpy ride.

- There will be a lot of scientific conjecture and theorizing which may someday prove incomplete or even wrong. Nevertheless, everything that I have written is the complete and unadulterated truth as I see it.

- I have a very curious mind. In my life, I have ventured fairly deeply down the "rabbit hole" for screenwriting, philosophy, history, and science, just to name a few topics. Jumping between these areas may generate some cognitive dissonance if you try to "pigeonhole" me, so I would ask that you just accept it from the start.

- Last but not least, you may wonder, "Is this guy trying to teach me something or sell me something?" Well, the answer is both! I am going to teach you what causes aging and disease and if you choose to, you can become one of my telomerase activation clients, purchase a home study course, or attend a seminar to participate more deeply.

In the spirit of open disclosure, I now draw open the Great and Powerful Oz's curtain and I will reveal to you, dear reader, my writing strategy, gleaned from years as a screenwriter.

There are eleven chapters in this book, each one logically following the other, like the scenes in a properly constructed movie.

You can expect every chapter to have one or two strong visual metaphors. "Show, don't tell" is the adage in screenwriting, and speaking of screenwriting, we will also reference some classic movie scenes to bring home some points along the way.

Every chapter will require an emotional investment from you, the reader. And finally, every chapter will have some kind of dilemma that will hopefully keep you turning the pages. A dilemma is the engine of any good story and usually involves an unanswered question because of a choice between two very good choices or two really bad choices.

So, without further ado, the dilemma of this first chapter is: "Why do we age and would it be morally wrong or punishable to stop it?

1

WHY DO WE GET OLD?

An error does not become truth by reason of multiplied propagation. Nor does truth become error because nobody sees it.

—Mohandas ("don't call me Mahatma") Gandhi

I like to ask questions. Always did, always will. I taught my sons that if you ask the question "why?" five times in a row, you will invariably run into these dreaded roadblocks to wisdom: "I don't know," "That's a silly question," or the dreaded "It just is." Go ahead and try it on the smartest person you know.

For example, "Why is the sky blue?" Because our atmosphere absorbs the other colors. But WHY? Because air particles scatter the non-blue light preferentially. WHY? Because light is a wave/particle phenomenon that appears to propagate through a medium in which there are other particles, and they interact. WHY? Because of the forces of electromagnetism and some other grand unified field stuff we haven't yet figured out. WHY? Because even with superconducting supercolliders and really cool theories, the model can't be tested and depends on a bunch of assumptions that are arbitrary. WHY? "Humph. It just is. Ask

God!" HA! Five questions and even Stephen Hawking is staring down checkmate.

Anyway, throughout my life as a student, teacher, physician, father, and citizen of this world, I have never stopped asking, "Why?"

I have learned (sometimes the hard way) that asking "why" often makes people upset. Yet, I can't seem to stop asking "stupid" questions until I reach one of the three stupid answers listed above.

The emotional investment of this chapter is that you are scared and should be scared of getting old, sick, losing your mind, suffering, and burdening your loved ones as you decay and eventually die. There it is. That is the elephant in every one of our rooms!

The visual metaphor I want you to have is the proverbial Emperor wearing his "new clothes" as I point out and shout, "But he's not wearing ANY clothes!"

What is this Thing We Call "Aging?"

Because we humans live amongst other humans of all ages, we are acutely aware of our own frailty and constantly reminded of the limited amount of time that we have in this existence. The passage of time and our own mortality undeniably are the central obsessions of our conscious and subconscious lives.

One of the critical functions of religion and mythology is to answer the question, "What will happen to me after I die?" Implicit in the question is the assumption that we are actually alive, and that we were created or born into this life. Of note, these basic assumptions are deemed false in some religions, such as Jainism, Hinduism, and Buddhism.

Just as we need to assume the existence of subatomic particles called bosons and immutable laws of physics in order to have a discussion about cosmology, we will concede to the illusion of *Samsara* (the Hindu concept of endless birth, life, death, and rebirth) and reject pantheism (the notion that everything is divine) and panpsychism (the notion that everything is consciousness).

The rules of our Western "common sense" reality presuppose that you and I are individual people and that our consciousness emerges from our physical body and mind (and possibly our soul). Our lives are the byproduct of sensory experiences that we process and the thoughts, beliefs, and actions that we generate within the field of physical reality, social reality, and our own self-generated reality. Mom and dad put egg and sperm together and we developed into a newborn baby, who grew up, has had some experience with illness and seeing others die, and is capable of reading this book.

Some people say God is the reason for everything. The unfortunate thing about any God theory is that it truly explains very little, and is quite easy-to-vary by simply replacing one god with any thousands of others that have been worshipped. So really, upper case "G-O-D" is the equivalent of a parent answering, "Because I said so" to every question a child might ask. A child raised like that could never learn to think on its own.

David Deutsch, an Oxford professor of physics, explains quite lucidly how science has always advanced in his wonderful TED talk delivered July of 2009 in Oxford, England. (TED is a group that sponsors self-consciously cool talks on Technology, Education, and Design). He points out that throughout mankind's history of philosophy, religion and science, only the pursuit of "hard-to-vary" explanations can lead to the immutable knowledge and understanding that we current endow our sciences with. This idea of the "hard-to-vary" explanation is one that we will revisit often in this book.

By the way, I respect everyone's beliefs but I don't believe that any one religion has a monopoly on truth any more than I think that a supreme deity has his sandals up on the couch rooting for Alabama's Crimson Tide every Saturday. I may already have alienated some people with that statement, so I'll go ahead and alienate some more with this proclamation: if you truly believe that God has ordained you to grow old and that there is nothing that you should do to resist it because it will jeopardize your good standing with God, then I suggest you stop reading this book.

Still reading? Good. As a movie from the 1970s suggested, "heaven can wait." So let's agree from the outset that safely and sanely resisting aging is a good thing and the reason we are still on the same page, literally and figuratively.

The next chapter reveals how my father's brain cancer compelled me to become interested in the topic of aging, but suffice it to say that my independent research (and that should conjure an image of me in my pajamas, late at night, on Wikipedia) uncovered about a half dozen popular theories that appeared to be science-based and which had their own staunch believers on a par with those in any monastery, mosque or temple.

I will present the other major theories of aging, but a telomere theory seemed the most reasonable to me. When I combined telomere biology with an understanding of stem cells, I came up with my own "Telomere/Stem Cell Theory of Aging." Don't worry if you don't understand all the concepts of the theory yet. You will by the end of the book.

Dr. Ed Park's Telomere/Stem Cell Theory of Aging
Following are axioms and corollaries of my Stem Cell Theory of Aging. Axioms are things we assume to be true and corollaries are statements that naturally flow from axioms.

Axiom 1: Because of the mechanics of copying DNA, telomeres always grow shorter with each cell division.

Axiom 2: Stem cells and Cancer cells (possible mutant stem cells) are capable of self-immortalizing by lengthening their telomeres as a result of activating telomerase.

> Corollary 2.1: Telomere lengths in the chromosomes of stem cells are dynamic and lengthen or shorten as a function of environmental effects, telomerase activation, chromosomal maintenance, and replicative burden.

> Corollary 2.2: Since T-cells of the cellular immune system are all stem-like in nature, senescence or aging of T-cells results in worsening immune function reflected in higher rates of infection and cancer.

Axiom 3: Differentiated, non-stem cells cannot be younger (telomere length) or healthier (genetic integrity) than their most recent stem cell progenitor.

Axiom 4: For non-stem cells, which can't utilize their telomerase, the Hayflick Limit is the cause of apoptosis ("programmed" cell death) and protects us from rogue cell lines that have acquired dangerous changes from DNA transcription errors, erroneous splicing, and oxidative or ionizing stresses.

Axiom 5: All dividing cells constantly monitor themselves for chromosomal damage but if immortal stem cells fail to undergo apoptosis and replacement with younger, better versions, the aging phenotype will manifest.

My Hypothesis: Aging is caused by accumulated DNA damage in stem cells, primarily caused by the shortening of their telomeres. If the stem cells' telomeres can be protected or altered by telomerase activation, then the effects of aging may be slowed and possibly reversed.

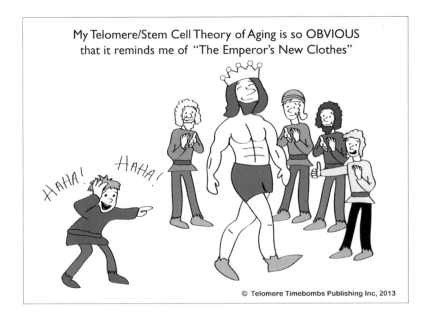

Some things are just obvious — like my theory of aging

This "Telomere/Stem Cell Theory of Aging" is the naked Emperor in his new clothes. Nothing in this theory, besides my final hypotheses, could be considered the least bit controversial in light of current science. This theory is literally the only thing that makes sense to me, is nearly impossible-to-vary, and it is so painfully obvious and logical that I don't really understand why nobody has stated it yet. Someday, people will read this book and say, "Duh. That's not a theory but merely a restatement of the obvious!" But before you accept that the only suit the emperor wears is the one given on his birthday, let us first praise and then bury the other theories once and for all.

Let's start with the first easy-to-vary and impossible-to-justify theory-- an *amuse-bouche* called the cancer theory. It states that aging was evolutionarily selected for in order to prevent the development of cancer. This theory bumps up against the human fossil record showing that it was nearly impossible for humans to ever to reach the advanced age at which cancer occurs. So how could evolution or natural selection take place if nobody ever lived long enough to develop cancer?

The main evolutionary theory of aging requires more consideration because it seems plausible at first. The logic goes something like this: the group, as a whole, benefits when older, post-reproductive individuals die off; so our species evolved a self-destruct mechanism (like the tapes that would self-destruct on Mr. Phelps in every *Mission Impossible* intro).

This evolutionary theory is a bit like the dystopian movie *Logan's Run* (MGM, 1976). In that classic science fiction story, because of the scarcity of resources in the post-apocalyptic future, everyone living in the safely domed city lived with the awareness that they had a "death-day" celebration at age 30 called "The Carousel." This is when they would voluntarily join other 30-year-olds in a ritualized public display of levitation, rapture, and explosion.

The problem with this theory is that evolution, as originally explained by Charles Darwin, takes place on an individual "survival of the fittest" level. So how can an individual be selected for genes that don't benefit the individual but benefit some abstract concept as "the greater good of my tribe?" Besides, how is rapid dying a survival benefit when male humans can reproduce well into their golden years?

Perhaps the salvation of the Evolutionary Theory of Aging lays in what evolutionary biologist Richard Dawkins called "the selfish gene?" Dawkins, an eminent scientist and thought leader, reduced the scale of evolution, proposing that genes (self-propagating DNA sequences) and memes (self-propagating ideas) are acting to preserve themselves. But he failed to elucidate a mechanism for this conscious or coordinated action. With all due respect to Dawkins, it might be said that the so-called "selfish gene" is itself a meme that is propagating far too extensively. We will learn in the next chapter that genes are nothing more than DNA sequences encoding for messenger RNA, which will be translated into a series of amino acids that form a discrete protein.

Why the jaundiced view of "selfish genes?" Because I cannot see how genes are players. Dawkins doesn't provide any clear and hard-to-vary explanation how they possess the agency to act selfishly, coordinate with other genes, dictate the ontogeny (the life course) of the host, and thereby contribute to the cosmic destiny of our species.

The "selfish gene" theory is a bit of sophistry akin to monkeys typing Shakespeare. To say a gene determines destiny is like saying the clarinet player in your high school orchestra created Beethoven's "Moonlight Sonata."

On the other hand, we will discuss in a later chapter the concept that cells, like our sperm and eggs, could rightly be considered selfish, because they have agency. In other words, their actions can be understood as selfish and competitive.

Another analogy: A fair election is not dictated by pamphlets or ideologies, but rather by the people who cast the votes. Similarly, most processes in the body are mediated at the cellular and especially the stem cell level of action. That is why cell nutrients are too small and lifestyle choices are too large in scale to provide any robust explanatory power.

In my years of learning from patients who are expert at due diligence when it comes to longevity, I find they take too many supplements and place too much emphasis on family history of diseases. Those factors are smaller and larger than the critical level of cellular agency. But until a telomerase activator was discovered to help preserve and replace stem cells, what else was available?

Returning now to a classic Darwinian evolutionary theory of aging, it simply goes against the selfishness of each individual's interests. The individual is trying to be the fittest and to survive the longest time possible, not "carousel" himself or herself out of existence. An evolutionary theory of aging provides no reasonable mechanism for how this evolved and doesn't address the presence of individual aging in non-social creatures across the animal kingdom.

So a "greater good," *Logan's Run* model of aging is not only easy-to-vary, its existence presupposes an intelligent, strategic designer. So this theory is theistic in nature, meaning it is god-based. Since god theories are the easiest-to-vary, we will dismiss them, thereby hopefully mollifying Richard Dawkins, the author of the anti-theistic *The God Delusion* (Mariner Books, 2008). Hopefully, he's not a fan of Alabama football.

The next aging theories are brought to us by the often oxymoronic "social sciences" and are easy-to-vary and hence, easy-to-dismiss. They include the "Activity and Continuity" theories suggesting that aging occurs because people become less active and fail to continue to do the things that kept them young, such as socializing and working. Talk about putting the cart before the horse!

Saying people "lose it because they don't use it" goes against everything we see from passionate adults and seniors who are engaged physically, professionally, emotionally and spiritually, but whose bodies continue to decay. The mind is willing but the body weakens.

The next interesting theory is one that we will revisit when we talk about apoptosis, or programmed cell death: namely mitochondrial dysfunction. Mitochondria are tiny bacteria that were incorporated into our cells during the course of evolution. Here again, I believe the cart is before the horse because the oxidative chemicals that leak out of the mitochondria when a cell is old may actually represent the cell's own attempt to self-destruct.

There is a theory called the "accumulative-waste theory" that is hopelessly vague and therefore hard to disprove. It states that something generally called "waste products" build up in cells and that is the cause of aging. In most cases, my Telomere/Stem Cell Theory of Aging would render that argument irrelevant, unless waste accumulation occurs at a preferentially irreversible rate in just our stem cells.

The final theories harmonize with my own theory. They include the "mis-repair theory" whereby the DNA damage is repaired incorrectly, the "somatic mutation theory" which states that damage to the genes of cells accumulates and causes aging, and finally the "error accumulation theory." All three of these theories merely state that genetic damage tends to accumulate over time and this is irrefutable.

When you compare the preceding theories with my Telomere/Stem Cell Theory of Aging, I believe mine is clearly the hardest-to-vary.

So let's just restate my theory in plain English:

It is an indisputable fact that there are special cells called stem cells that are responsible for making nearly infinite copies of themselves as a mother cell and a more differentiated daughter cell. The daughter cells, unable to immortalize themselves like their stem cell mother because they lack telomerase activity, eventually burn through their telomeres and die off. This is actually a good thing preventing us from becoming giant starving blobs.

But telomerase activity naturally preserves and protects the stem cells to some degree. Despite our attempts to bolster telomerase activity through healthy lifestyle choices, stem cells acquire mutations from telomere shortening that manifest as the clinical signs, symptoms, and diseases associated with aging. Genetic damage is mostly recognized by the stem cells themselves and they kill themselves off. But over the course of a lifetime, more and more little problems arise and even the quality of the replacement stem cells deteriorates.

It really is just that simple.

The Hidden Script: "It's Too Good to be True"

Let us now switch gears completely and discuss whether it is morally wrong to want to stay young and healthy. In a word, no. If that were the case, then organized religion would frown upon exercise, healthy eating, sleep, stress reduction, and seeing a doctor.

People have always wanted to stay healthy and live longer. One of the most ancient archetypes of our storytelling has been this pursuit of eternal youth. From Gilgamesh, to Dr. Faust, to Count Dracula, no one ever succeeds without paying a price. Cheating death is just "too good to be true".

Most storytelling seems to imply that you can't have something you yearn for without a wish backfiring on you, whether it be King Midas' touch of gold, "The Gift of The Magi," or basically every Twilight Zone episode ever made. "Be careful what you wish for" is the tenacious subtext that I have to overcome when I explain telomerase activation medicine. Somewhere deep down, the knee-jerk fear of people is that if you try to live longer, you'll get more cancer, grow a tail, or will just be too frail to enjoy the extra years.

But wait! The forbidden promise of living longer, even eternally, is right there in the Book of Genesis from the Bible. Many people don't know this, but there were really two trees in the Garden of Eden. The first tree was the Tree of Knowledge (of good and evil) and the second tree was the Tree of Eternal Life.

Here is the relevant passage from the Bible:

"Then the LORD God said, "Behold, the man has become like one of us in knowing good and evil. Now, lest he reach out his hand and take also of the tree of life and eat, and live forever—"therefore the LORD God sent him out from the garden of Eden to work the ground from which he was taken."

— *English Standard Version,* Genesis 3:22

The antediluvian (a fancy word for before the flood) patriarchs like Noah and Methuselah lived into their tenth centuries. But God decided that human life expectancy needed to be shortened to 70 years just before sending the flood to engulf mankind.

Since leaving the Garden of Eden, humanity has grown up considerably. Maybe we are ready for the car keys? We have built civilizations, explanatory systems, commerce, art, and a culture allowing me to sit down and write this book so millions of people can potentially read and understand it just a few months later.

If I'm correct and we now possess the ability to keep our stem cells young and healthy by activating telomerase, then perhaps we have figuratively gotten ourselves back to the Garden and God will allow for a new covenant by resetting our biological clocks.

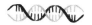

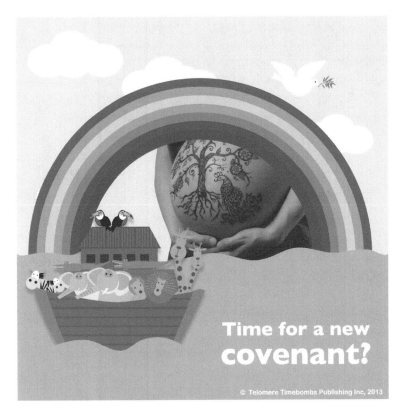

Time for a new
covenant?

© Telomere Timebombs Publishing Inc, 2013

Will humanity soon recapture its lost longevity?

As you read on, you must decide whether it is morally wrong to live a longer and healthier life. But I caution you: don't let the false doctrine of "too good to be true" be the sole determinant.

The truth is that everything about our lives is improbable and much too good to be true. In Buddhism, there is the doctrine of the "The Preciousness of Human Birth." You were the only one of 20 million sperm to "score" with the egg. You have already won a lottery! Your soul wasn't born on an inhospitable planet or into the body of a fruit fly, so really, life is pretty darn good for you and me, don't you think?

As the philosopher Arthur Schopenhauer said, "truth goes through several stages: first it is ignored, then it is ridiculed, and then it is deemed to be self-evident."

And just because you and I are among the early adopters of the truth that aging is now a choice rather than a curse, believe me when I say the other 7 billion of our fellow souls will be joining this party fairly soon.

But before you let such matters of life and death and your eternal soul weigh too heavily upon you, let me share the story of how I came to write this book for you.

2

MY HERO'S JOURNEY

"There is a saying in Tibetan, 'Tragedy should be utilized as a source of strength.' No matter what sort of difficulties, how painful experience is, if we lose our hope, that's our real disaster."

— Lhamo (they call me the Dalai Lama) Dondrub

George Lucas, while creating *Star Wars,* relied heavily upon the work of mythologist Joseph Campbell, who in turn borrowed heavily from the work of Swiss psychiatrist and mystic, Carl Jung. Campbell was a lifelong student of mythology and comparative religion. When anyone first learns to construct and deconstruct stories these days, they learn the so-called "monomyth," or what Campbell termed the archetypal "hero's journey."

In order to create structure from the ashes of my chaotic life, the subheadings of this chapter will borrow from this hero's journey structure. For more information, check out Bill Moyers' amazing PBS documentary interview series and book featuring Joseph Campbell called *The Power of Myth* (Anchor, 1991). The diagram that follows is an illustration of my life seen through this model of the one story told over and over again.

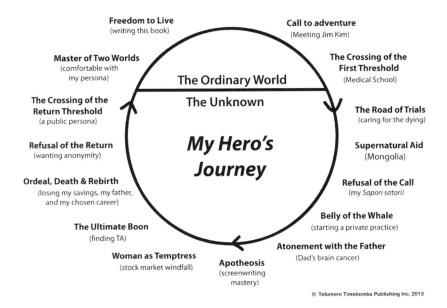

My "hero's journey" thus far

Plot Synopsis for my Life

An altruistic and idealistic young man plans to save the world as an international public health doctor but his dreams are abandoned under pressure from family. He makes and then loses a fortune, his career is destroyed by a government plot, and he loses his father to brain cancer. But his rising spirit and hidden forces lead him to a rebirth and the discovery of the elixir that will truly accomplish what he set out to do: to save the world.

The Ordinary World

I was born the third and final child of two Korean immigrants who were living and working in Saskatchewan, Canada in the year 1967. They both escaped North Korea between World War II and the Korean War but met in the United States in 1962 when my mother was working as a nurse and my father was training as a physician.

My mother was what they now refer to as a "tiger mom" and was not the least bit subtle about declaring medicine to be the preordained calling of her three children. My eldest sister, Ann, squeamish at the sight of blood but giddy in the presence of a thesaurus, became the black sheep of the family with her choice of law as a career.

My brother, Ronald, would have loved to be a "dot.com" pioneer and surf bum but he somehow did manage to fulfill his "tiger mom" programming and became a physician. For some time, my mother basked in the glory of sending all three of her children to Harvard College, which for Asian-Americans would roughly be the equivalent of being Peyton and Eli Manning's dad in mainstream American culture.

The Call to Adventure

When I was in high school, I first met another Asian associated with Harvard, Jim Kim, who was a medical student at the time. We met while playing volleyball at a Korean-American youth camp in the mountains of Southern California. I got so excited about the sport that when I returned to school, a friend and I founded the high school volleyball team that still thrives thirty years later.

While still in high school, I met Jim again while taking summer school classes at UCLA. I still vividly recall sitting at lunch listening to Jim explain his aspirations to study medical anthropology and work in the field of international public health. I became one of many people who recall meeting Jim, feeding off his passion, and wanting to grow up to be just like him.

Jim fulfilled that dream and much more as a professor at Harvard's Medical and Public Health Schools, as the director of HIV/AIDS initiatives for the World Health Organization, as the President of Dartmouth University, and now as the President of the World Bank.

My call to adventure was planted there by Jim Kim and manifested at Harvard College as a pre-med/anthropology major. I did public health work in Ecuador and found I was never more alive than when immersed in a foreign culture and working toward improving the health and lives of people who could benefit from education and tools of self-reliance.

During my junior year at Harvard, I researched female circumcision, the ritual genital cutting practiced in some parts of Africa, and had arranged to travel to war-torn Eritrea to do field research on those practices. The thought of living in trenches while Soviet-made helicopter gunships flew above probably should have concerned me but it didn't. Unfortunately, a hotel bombing in Khartoum and the resulting deaths of British foreign aid workers caused a cancellation of my visa from the Eritrean People's Liberation Front so that call to adventure was never fulfilled.

Crossing the Threshold

My second mentor was Dr. Allan Rosenfield, the dean of the Columbia School of Public Health. I chose medical school at

Columbia College of Physicians and Surgeons in New York City because in only four years, I could earn both my medical doctor and my master of public health degrees while studying with Allan.

Allan had lived my dream life as a public health physician and even raised kids while working around the world, mainly in Thailand, as a researcher in family planning and a trained Ob-Gyn.

After Allan's fieldwork in Asia and Africa, he returned to become the director of the international family planning non-profit organization known as The Population Council. That organization invented and reintroduced a "Copper-T" intrauterine device (IUD) after the litigation surrounding the infamous Dalkon Shield had for many years rendered the IUD unavailable in the United States. As a 99% effective, reversible, non-hormonal method of birth control, the IUD is even more perfectly suited for women with limited health care access in developing countries. It is the gold standard for appropriate contraceptive technology and the most frequently used method worldwide. Why? Because of its simplicity and because the moral and intellectual property rights to make this simple device of copper, plastic, and a fishing line were given away freely around the world by Allan's Population Council long ago.

Class action litigation and the lack of corporate profits (a theme we will explore in Chapter 10: "The Medical-industrial complex"), had killed the IUD but Allan's research and his organization's philanthropy resurrected the little cross upon which I would later be crucified.

After graduation with my MD and Masters in Public Health in 1993, I kept in touch with Dr. Rosenfield because he returned annually to my Ob-Gyn residency program at Harvard Medical

School's Beth Israel Hospital to honor his father, the former chief of staff.

After my first year of residency, I married. After completing four years of residency, and in preparation for what I thought was going to be a career in international aid and development, I took a job at staff model HMO called Kaiser Permanente in Orange County, California while I studied for my board exams and collected a lifetime's worth of clinical experience.

Truthfully, Ob-Gyn is probably the only medical specialty I am suited for because it is a happy field in which good medicine is rewarded with a happy ending: a healthy baby!

Countertransference is when a doctor becomes emotionally entangled with their patient and I suffer from a strong case of it. I am very empathic so if I can't cure someone, it makes me very unhappy and I take any worsening of their health quite hard and quite personally.

The Road of Trials (Initiation)
I will now tell you three stories about cases that helped shape my view of medicine as disease management and why I am not cut out for it. These stories put into perspective why I am so grateful that telomerase activation medicine has given me the opportunity to truly help people and feel uplifted as a result.

I will never forget my very first night in a hospital as a third year medical student. It was at Columbia's Allen Pavilion during my surgical rotation. That morning, as bright-eyed and bushy-tailed medical students and residents, we had rounded on this smiling lovely lady who had undergone intestinal surgery for

Crohn's disease, a chronic, often progressive disease affecting the intestines.

I could not have imagined that before dawn, I would be sitting on top of her, performing chest compressions in a radiology suite, and watching the life ebb from her frightened eyes. Chest compressions! And the sound of cracking ribs, agonal gas and feces passing from below and above, and all the while, the anesthesiologist cursing the stool splattering on all of us as she struggled to mechanically ventilate the patient with a hand-held bag.

There is a light of life in the eyes and when it left her as she died, it was both sublime and disturbing.

Did I cause her genetic disease? No. Did I do her surgery? No. Didn't I try my best to resuscitate her? Yes. Then why did I feel so awful? So guilty?

My Harlem Hospital pediatrics rotation was during the height of the crack cocaine and AIDS epidemic in New York City. I had always wanted to be a pediatrician, but the experience of drawing blood at 4AM from an screaming 7-year-old orphan with AIDS brought home how real countertransference felt to me. He had no idea why he was suffering and my actions, although for his own good, seemed to only to deepen his pain.

My bleakest experience with the vanity and futility of modernized hospital care came as an intern on my internal medicine rotation at Beth Israel. One of my patients was Charlie, a young man dying of AIDS before the effective drug therapies for HIV were invented. For weeks, I administered a list of ineffective drugs with their own awful side effects to Charlie as his consciousness waned, largely from the dissolving of his brain by a viral infection. I felt so helpless as I watched all his organs fail amidst the opportunistic infections that were overwhelming his once beautiful, but now emaciated frame. In his late twenties, he looked like he was 100, perfectly illustrating what I would later come to realize: that AIDS is simply aging of the immune system and that aging is a form of acquired immune deficiency.

I had the pleasure of knowing Charlie and a bit of his light while he was still somewhat present. It was notably the first and last time I prescribed marijuana pills. They were given to help his appetite. But make no mistake; Charlie was going to die in pain, inexorably, and without dignity. The last week of his life, I was providing "comfort care," which was really a euphemism for giving him increasing doses of morphine that placed him deeper into a stupor and decreased his capacity and desire to breathe.

I'll never forget sitting at his bedside, watching him. Many times I thought he had just died. Charlie would stop breathing for an impossibly long 20 or 30 seconds, and then, he gasped yet another deep, shuddering breath. This went on for days despite my administering an increasing dose of morphine drip every morning on my daily rounds.

His consciousness had already been destroyed by a virus called CMV so why did the medical-industrial complex have us keeping his body alive for so long? Why did we prolong his agony? In the end, this macabre spectacle, an undignified and pointless end to a beautiful life, was costly to society, painful to his loved ones, and had a very personal impact on me: it eradicated my own interest in caring for terminally ill people.

In stark contrast to my experience with CPR on a dying woman, torturing a scared orphan, and presiding over the comfort care of an end stage AIDS patient, my experience with Ob-Gyn was blissful and fulfilling. After fourteen years of practicing clinical medicine, delivering babies and doing routine well-woman care, I can literally count on one hand the number of times I felt regret or hopelessness from caring for my patients.

My dreams of becoming a public health physician were on schedule and while in my fourth and final year at Kaiser, I traveled to El Salvador on behalf of the US Agency for International Development to promote IUD usage among doctors and nurse practitioners there. Together with Professor Lara from Mexico City, we spent three days leading a seminar for women's health providers invited from every corner of that country.

In a fascinating case study of medical anthropology, in Mexico, the Population Council's Copper-T IUD is used routinely in the majority of women because it costs very little to make, requires no compliance, and is reversible. Right next door, in El Salvador, patients and providers alike almost never use the IUD because they wrongly believed it instigated abortion and caused birth defects. While I was there, I actually met doctors who, in order to deter IUD use, confessed to inventing stories of babies being born with IUD's embedded in their foreheads or holding them like vampire hunters.

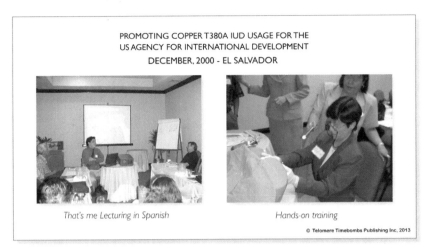

PROMOTING COPPER T380A IUD USAGE FOR THE
US AGENCY FOR INTERNATIONAL DEVELOPMENT
DECEMBER, 2000 - EL SALVADOR

That's me Lecturing in Spanish   *Hands-on training*

© Telomere Timebombs Publishing Inc, 2013

Promoting IUD usage in El Salvador

While working with the Salvadoran government officials, I was allowed to review maternal mortality statistics. I was saddened to learn that suicide was the major cause of death because young women, afraid of the shame of bearing a child out of wedlock, killed themselves. Having a hidden and effective method of contraception surely could have saved many lives. The opportunity to use my IUD expertise, language fluency, and public health experience was wonderful and I knew that I had chosen the right path for my career.

Supernatural Aid

When I returned, Allan put me in contact with an opportunity to be the family planning director for the entire country of Mongolia, as he had done in Thailand. From Pap smears in Orange County to the policy maker for an entire country? I was ecstatic. "Finally!" I thought. Twelve years training and thousands of hours of clinical experience were going to pay off. Whether living in a yurt or a bleak socialist concrete tenement, it was going to be an adventure of a lifetime.

Refusal of the Call

Little did I know that I was about to have another life-changing restaurant chat on par with meeting Jim Kim fourteen years before. Faced with the probability of living in Mongolia, my wife and the mother of our then two-year-old son summoned my mother and father to sit me down in an Italian restaurant called Sapori in order to perform a vocational intervention. It just now occurs to me that the restaurant's name was just a heartbeat, or in EKG terms, a QRS electrical complex, away from satori, or a moment of Zen enlightenment. My satori at Sapori was to discover that my life course had already been laid out, in no uncertain terms, by my mom, dad, and spouse. They all read me the riot act about being a serious person and giving up dreams of saving the world or doing anything else out of the ordinary.

I was not pleased. Despite our plans to travel the world with kids in tow, like the Rosenfields had done in Thailand, it seems that my dreams of international public health medicine were subject to group familial veto. And so it came to pass that the need to be respectable and normal trumped my ambitions of becoming the next Jim Kim or Allan Rosenfield.

Who knows what would have been had I gone that route? But in 2001, I decided to hang a shingle and become a solo private practice doctor in the suburbs because HMO medicine by committee, paid by the hour, was not suited for my countertransference-prone, high-output style of practicing medicine.

Belly of the Whale

Building a practice from nothing was a challenge at first but having my own hours, patients, and the expansion of my practice into cosmetic procedures such as laser, Botox™ and other skin fillers kept me moving forward professionally and economically. Thankfully, my parents were able to loan the practice enough money to purchase the lasers. However, this financial enabling established a precedent that would later haunt our family when circumstances became desperate.

Atonement with the Father

I first became interested in aging the moment my father was diagnosed with brain cancer in 2004. My dad's greatest joy in life was learning so this was a particularly cruel sentence and, given the fact that he had been healthy his whole life, it seemed very unjust. The thought of my father dying put me into an early midlife tailspin.

The next two years, my family and I deferred to doctors who could only give false hope for his affliction. They advised and we agreed to have him cut, burned, and poisoned, destroying that beautiful mind and body until he drew his final breath. When he passed, I was holding his hand, noting the surprise and fear in his gaze like my Crohn's patient, but unlike my AIDS patient, Charlie, there was not to be any next gasp for air.

If you have ever had a loved one die from cancer, you know the bleak death march you are coerced into walking. Is it all just so the doctors can feel good about what they are doing or to support some drug company research? My faith that there has to be a better way led to the righteous indignation I have outlined in Chapter 10: "The Medical-industrial complex."

Apotheosis

As you might have predicted from reading the first chapter, the sudden awareness of death prompted me to ask the question "why do we age?" So, at the age of 36, I began to seriously investigate why people get old and sick. That led to my Telomere/Stem Cell Theory of Aging and my first screenplay idea.

The specter of my own insignificance and frailty forced me to conclude that life was too short to do a relatively easy and predictable job, like being a doctor. So I decided my true calling was to be a screenwriter. Really, as the cliché goes, I wanted to direct but I didn't discover that until years later.

So I passionately dedicated myself to learning the craft of writing for two solid years. If there was a book, lecture or a video on the subject, I devoured it. I watched all the great movies and many of the mediocre ones too. And I wrote, edited, submitted, and pitched my work to Hollywood producers. When did I have time to do this? I eliminated television from my mind's diet and studied and wrote after the kids went to sleep every night and well into the wee hours of the morning.

My first screenplay, Maximum Lifespan, that I later adapted into a graphic novel, is a sci-fi thriller in which an unscrupulous scientist named Ken Garrett clones himself into genetically-engineered clones, who believe they are sons, and then tries to download his consciousness into their bodies to cheat death and live forever.

The story began as a thought experiment about what kind of world it would be if people had the power to stop aging with telomerase activation. What were people capable of in the name of extending their lives? What problems would arise? Would only the wealthy have access? Can consciousness be stored in and transferred from a machine?

Interestingly, many things in that story have since come true. When I wrote it, I had no idea that Cal Harley, the Chief Science Officer of the massive Geron Corporation of Menlo Park, had already found a telomerase-activating needle in the haystack of candidate molecules, and that human testing had already begun. In my story, Dr. Ken Garrett wins a Nobel Prize for telomerase activation. In the real world, the Nobel Prize in 2009 was awarded for the same discovery.

My story features pet cloning, which became commercially available in 2008 and oddly enough, licensed by the Geron Corporation. And finally, avatar-based adult interactive entertainment, used for transfer of the evil Ken's consciousness to his cloned sons, is an ongoing and expanding real world technology. If you want to learn more about tomorrow's technologies today, check out my prophetic, 191-page full-color graphic novel. Maximum Lifespan (Pileus Productions, 2010). It is available for purchase at my website at www.maximumlifespancomic.com, from Barnes & Noble stores (extremely rare for a self-published book) and also as an iTunes download.

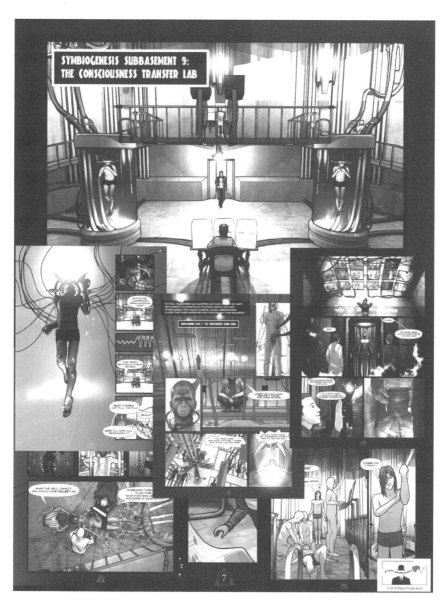

Pages from my graphic novel, *Maximum Lifespan*

Before I stopped writing to focus on telomerase activation medicine, I wrote another comic screenplay called *Manchild*, a teleplay for "House MD", and created my favorite screenplay, *Hypatia (aka Nike's Last Stand)*. That was a historical epic that won an award at the 2007 Houston Film Festival. It is about the real life philosopher and human rights martyr, Hypatia, who lived in 4th century Alexandria, Egypt.

Woman as Temptress (or material temptations)

Over the previous years, I had enjoyed a long run of successful stock option trading with the greatest windfall from stock options around the kitschy plastic shoes known as Crocs®. For one nanosecond around my 40th birthday, I had amassed over 10 million dollars in my bank account. That proved to be a problem because I thought I was bulletproof and we ended up spending and living as though there would never be any worries about money again. How wrong we were.

The Ultimate Boon

After my successful options trading windfall, I was surfing the internet in the fall of 2007 when I stumbled upon the existence of Geron's telomerase activator, TA-65®. Because of my recent windfall, the trip to New York and the $25,000 required to become the 19th person the world to ingest TA-65 didn't deter me. We will further discuss the provenance of TA-65 in Chapter 8: "Telomerase activators."

So in the fall of 2007, I flew out to New York after being permitted to read all the safety and efficacy data on TA-65. There, I met with Noel Patton, the founder of T.A. Sciences®. Noel seemed very honest and passionate about his product, although he did question why a 39-year-old would want to take an anti-aging pill.

Having done my due diligence, I could not be deterred despite the package warning not to take TA-65 at my age. After starting it, I honestly didn't feel much. Weighing in at 200 pounds and 5' 10", I was obese, with high blood pressure, fatty liver, high cholesterol, and low testosterone. But after three months, despite not changing my diet or exercising, I had lost 15 pounds, mostly around my visceral belly fat. I had a new improved outlook on life and a greatly improved outward appearance, although it was only a year after my father had succumbed to brain cancer.

Because the idea of taking a pill to get younger might have sounded a bit crazy, I didn't tell anyone. But my patients, at their annual physicals, never failed to remark upon how I looked like a completely different person. They would rhetorically ask "what are you taking?" but if I actually tried to explain that I was taking and anti-aging pill, they would laugh.

To this day, I receive angry emails and Facebook® comments which are really rhetorical accusations, to the effect of "you mean to tell me you didn't change your diet or exercise at all?" And "why do you tell people you eat fast food if you are into healthy anti-aging?" I have been counseled to pretend that I did in fact change my diet and start exercising because that would set a better example, but it just wouldn't be true.

So how could taking a pill that is a telomerase activator cause a reversal in aging to occur? That will be the subject of Chapter 9: "Telomerase Activation Medicine."

After a year of hearing the backhanded compliment of "You look so good that I didn't recognize you!" I decided to ask if I could offer TA-65 to my own patients. That would cost me another $50,000 for the privilege of selling it and purchasing the testing equipment to measure biomarkers of aging, but luckily the windfall from my stock investing had not been squandered or lost...yet.

So in late 2008, I hung up a shingle and a few dozen souls found me and began the TA-65 journey with me as their Sherpa guide, if you will. Despite some local television news stories and an interview I did for Spanish language TV network, Telemundo, I did not have many patients until the Nobel Prize for telomerase activation in 2009 brought attention to the fact that the body already has the secret to eternal youth in every stem cell.

From my personal experience and the experiences of my earliest, pioneering patients, I believed TA-65 worked and was safe. I was having great results but both patients and I had real trouble believing, attributing, and understanding what was going on. It would take years of follow-ups, phone calls, and preparing for live webinars until I began to develop the clinical expertise I needed to confidently advise my patients.

But the wheel of fortune was about to take me down hard. After the financial crisis of 2008, people stopped having babies and cosmetic procedures and it was becoming impossible to hang on. Despite being the very first and one of the busiest doctors prescribing TA, it was three years before I ever made a profit selling it.

I was at a crossroads and my options were running out as fast as mortgage payments and maxed-out credit cards could drain them.

Speaking of options, I got very carried away with investing in stock options in the Geron Corporation, and my portfolio imploded like a neutron star. I suppose that a person's strengths are also their weaknesses. For me, my history of success with large options trades and my unwavering faith in telomerase activation were my downfall. Little did I know, the wheel of fortune could take me even lower.

Ordeal, Death and Rebirth

The final straw that should have broken this camel's back came from a health care fraud conviction that played out from 2008-2010. My expertise and first-hand knowledge of Mexican Copper-T IUDs led me to purchase generic ones from Mexico. I had been told by another physician that I respected that the use of generic, imported IUDs was a common practice in my community for those few of us willing to serve medically-indigent women without health insurance.

Understand that these Mexican IUDs were sterilely manufactured in United States FDA-registered factories under the license granted to them by Allan Rosenfield's Population Council. In fact, the Copper-T380A is the most used form of birth control globally because the intellectual property rights to produce it generically were granted to health care ministries worldwide and then sublicensed to private medical device manufacturers

Because the non-for-profit Population Council intended women to have a safe and affordable option for contraception, the exact same item only cost a few dollars each in Tijuana whereas the identical US one cost us about $300 dollars each to purchase from the sole American manufacturer. Inexplicably, our government's Medicaid program would reimburse doctors just $260 so we were forced into a situation in which we lost money every transaction but had to make it up in volume (as the joke goes).

Over the course of three years, I placed less than twenty of these into Medicaid patients, but the American distributor and the government had already resolved to set into motion a sort of "Sting" operation to go after me and other colleagues.

When a nurse from the Department of Health Services called to ask me whether I had used a generic IUD, it never even occurred to me that this would have been illegal. I welcomed them into my office for an audit and never thought to consult an attorney. Just as people sometimes purchase Canadian prescription drugs and just as I had known many patients who were instructed by fertility specialists to purchase extremely costly fertility vials from Mexico for use in American clinics, I thought there was no ethical or legal dilemma at all.

Later, I learned that the government prosecutors gave amnesty to doctors who were using Canadian-sourced IUDs which seemed a bit arbitrary.

As a result of the criminal charges filed against me, I was fined, advised to plead guilty to a misdemeanor charge of Medicare fraud for using a misbranded device, and served 100 hours of community service. After a year, the plea was withdrawn as if the offense had never occurred and the Medical Board did not sanction me.

I thankfully managed to emerge without any legal or medical board blemishes, but the conviction had the effect of excluding me from Medicare participation, which then precluded me from all hospital admissions and insurance plan participation. It was the equivalent of nuclear Armageddon for my ability to practice Ob-Gyn for at least five years.

Refusal of the Return

I am a very introverted person and I always felt uncomfortable trying to "sell" anyone on the benefits of TA. When I explain about a pill to reverse aging, most people I know just roll their eyes or mock me. I think that is sad because it not only is a prejudgment about my abilities and honesty but it is also a kind of negation of their own significance; what are the chances this Ed they know is at the epicenter of something so mindboggling?

I knew if I were going to help get the word out, it would mean becoming a public figure and evangelist. That was something I wasn't prepared to do, but I was borrowing money from relatives, and the money was going out but not coming in, and everything I tried in the stock market was a disaster. I see now that my inability to practice orthodox medicine was the Universe's way of burning my boats, like the Conquistador Cortés did to discourage thoughts of returning to Spain before the mission was done.

So I resolved to relinquish my anonymity for the greater good, and to pay the mortgage. I even took acting and musical theater classes to try to conquer my fear of speaking in front of people.

The Crossing of the Return Threshold
Whenever a few patients reported the same improvements, or in the case of rare and interesting changes, I would put together a live webinar and then produce a video complete with disease explanations, case reports, and live questions and answers. To date, there have been 45 of these webinars on topics ranging from high blood pressure, to insomnia, to Lyme Disease. The webinars alone represent over 1500 hours of work to make 1.2 days' worth of content. You can check them out on my website, www.RechargeBiomedical.com or from my YouTube channel, "drpark65."

Master of Two Worlds
After taking TA-65 for two years, I had continued to enjoy better health and my patients also were having dramatic

improvements. I was a complete believer but the Nobel Prize alone wasn't enough to grow the patient base.

Luckily, in 2010, Harvard research scientists showed that activation of telomerase could reverse aging in mice. Now there was the in vivo (meaning in real animals) proof of principle that some people needed before taking the leap of faith.

Things got so bad financially that in 2010, I couldn't afford to take TA-65 myself! But for the nine months that I didn't take it, I didn't feel any different and didn't put on any weight, leading me to conclude that the dysfunctional stem cells in my visceral fat had been vanquished for good. Interestingly, my telomeres did grow dramatically shorter during that time (I believe from stress and non-ingestion of TA-65) but the good news was I didn't shrivel up like a vampire at dawn's first light.

From 2010 to 2011, I worked hard to create more videos from case studies and grow a social media presence on Facebook, Twitter, iTunes, and YouTube. I did interviews for *Yahoo! Shine, Men's Journal, Vogue,* and I traveled to give lectures around the country about my theory of aging and clinical experiences to anti-aging conferences, wellness festivals, and at UCLA's Gerontology Research Group.

Freedom to Live

Why didn't I despair? Well, as hopeless as I got financially, I was being inspired by my TA patients and their stories of transformational change. I'd like to share one particular type of call that happens about once a week on average and it is as beautiful as hearing a newborn baby draw its first breath.

A patient who has been taking TA for a few weeks will call me from an airport or after a high school reunion and tell me "doc, all I can see is aging on these other people and I realize that now I can start all kinds of new projects. It's a game changer and I'm looking forward to so many things!"

Earlier, I explained how my empathic countertransference makes me avoidant of sick people. I don't do well with remorse and hopelessness. So now I like to say I'm still an obstetrician at heart; I just attend rebirths now. And the souls that I deliver back into the world are just slightly older than the ones I used to assist.

People are funny. The majority of my patients, after stopping and restarting a couple of times, do believe that TA-65 works and is a justifiable "cost of living well" expense, but they are unable to convince their spouses, friends, and relatives of its value even after being accused of plastic surgery or other hormonal manipulations to become younger. If I had to guess, I would say one of my "true believer" patients will tell 20 people about me and what they're taking and perhaps only five of those 20 will even bother to even look it up. Of those five people, the number of people that will actually invest the time to learn, watch my videos, and research online is very nearly zero.

As more prominent businessmen, athletes, and entertainers who currently take telomerase activators come out of the "TA closet" that number will increase dramatically. But starting to take TA because of the endorsement of a famous celebrity is the other side of the coin of rejecting TA because they haven't yet heard of it yet. I wrote this book so that people won't be fooled by paid celebrity-endorsements of false telomerase activators or multi-level marketing schemes because I'm sure they will be rampant very soon.

We all know that a celebrity endorsement is expensive but thankfully in the internet age, knowledge is free, however true understanding and wisdom is always earned so let us take the next three chapters to pay our dues and arm you with the tools to truly understand what is at the heart of disease and aging.

3

WHAT IS A TELOMERE?

"The curse of mortality. You spend the first portion of your life learning, growing stronger, more capable. And then, through no fault of your own, your body begins to fail. You regress. Strong limbs become feeble, keen senses grow dull, hardy constitutions deteriorate. Beauty withers. Organs quit. You remember yourself in your prime, and wonder where that person went. As your wisdom and experience are peaking, your traitorous body becomes a prison."

— Brandon Mull, <u>Fablehaven</u> (Aladdin, 2007)

Telomeres are timebombs on the end of every chromosome; hence the title of this book! Perhaps a better way to visualize would be to consider them burning fuses at both ends of a firecracker.

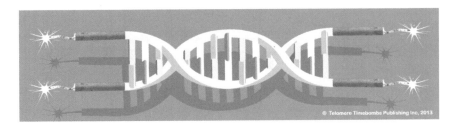

Telomeres are like burning fuses at the tips of chromosomes

We know that when the fuse reaches the firecracker, bad things happen. Likewise, when the telomeres in your stem cells burn too low, your genetic library becomes fragmented and recombined in unnatural ways.

The idea of billions of your chromosomes exploding daily might fill you with fear. Don't let it! As we will learn, it is an essential part of how our systems function properly.

The Central Dogma of Molecular Biology

Think of a chromosome as two very long text messages running in opposite directions. When I say long, I'm talking 50-200 million letters. Each of our 23 chromosomes has over 1,000 genes, or smaller segments, that encode for proteins, but these actual genes that encode "information" account for only 2% of the DNA and there are other many other poorly understood areas for controlling the expression of those genes and the form and function of the cell.

The "text" of the message consists of one of four distinct DNA molecules that we will call A,G,C and T. So a DNA chain, or chromosome, can be read as GATTACA, or whatever, 100 million times. It is a rule that the A type always pairs with the T type on the opposite, or complimentary, strand side. So let's say that in the diagram above, A is the red and T is the green. Do you see how they pair up? Likewise, a G always pairs with a C, and those would be the yellow and blue DNA molecules. Each rung of the chromosome's double helical ladder is what is known as a "base pair" and the base pair is the unit of length measurement to which we will refer when we discuss telomere lengths later. One entire chromosome might be 100 million base pairs but the telomere tips or burning fuses, are a maximum of about 15,000 base pairs in length in humans.

So unless there is a typographical error, one side precisely dictates how the other side, or its complimentary strand, must be assembled. Together, they are like a zipper. One strand consists of "the sense" and the other is just the other half of the zipper and is known as the "anti-sense" strand.

Without the unzipping and the precise assembly of complimentary strands, a process known as DNA replication, one mother cell could never divide into two daughters.

All life, I repeat, ALL life on this planet uses this exact same genetic coding language of DNA. Each gene is a discrete short sequence that can be transcribed into what is called messenger RNA. Messenger RNA, like the paper in a fortune cookie, emerges from the nucleus of a cell and is fed into micromachines called ribosomes, which translate each three "letter" RNA message into the appropriate next amino acid in that protein, which is just a chain of amino acids.

If it takes three letters to encode an amino acid, then a gene encoding a protein with 100 amino acids would need to be at least 300 base pairs long. Get it?

Let's say the DNA message is "GTT." The messenger RNA would have to read "CAA." That CAA tells the ribosome that the next amino acid will be glutamine. The assembly of a chain of amino acids makes what we know as a protein and depending on the amino acid sequences, they predictably fold into shapes that will dictate their form and function in the body. Scientists call the process of transcription and subsequent translation from the gene's DNA, into the messenger RNA, and finally into the gene's specific protein, the "central dogma of molecular biology."

By some inexplicable miracle, this same process takes place IN ALL LIFE ON THIS PLANET. Somehow, this process dictates cellular development and cooperation and results in amazing things from dragonflies to concert cellists when it occurs in stepwise and orchestrated fashion (pun intended).

So now that you understand the basics, let's ask a question: "Why do we have telomeres?" The answer is because our chromosomes are long and linear, not short and circular. I will explain by describing "less evolved" life forms that we call bacteria.

The Eukaryotic Revolution
Although bacteria use the same genetic machinery, they are each loners, or single cell organisms that possess only a miniscule circular chromosome. Bacterial chromosomes easily reproduce like one soap bubble becoming two soap bubbles and they don't have

telomeres. There aren't any tips to protect with telomeres because a circle has no ends. That is also why bacteria (also known as "prokaryotes" or "before the kernel") don't need a cell nucleus that protects their precious genetic library like our eukaryotic cells do. Eukaryotes comes from the Greek for "good kernel" or "good nut" meaning those cells have a nucleus.

About 1.5 billion years ago on this planet, it is thought that some bacteria became incorporated into protozoan cells in a process known as symbiogenesis. "Genesis" means the creation of new life and "symbio" is short for symbiosis, or the interdependence of two distinct species for their mutual survival. This eukaryotic revolution was pivotal for the evolution of more complicated life forms on earth.

In plants, those bacterial helpers contain chlorophyll and are known as chloroplasts. They convert sunlight into energy by photosynthesis. In animal cells, the bacteria that were incorporated are now known as mitochondria and they use chemical reactions to power our cells.

Having a nucleus, like a protected bubble inside the bubble of the cell itself, allowed for the development of extremely long and elaborate genetic libraries that we know as discrete chromosomes. In humans, we have 22 pairs (one set from mom and one set from dad) and the 23rd pair is known as the "sex chromosomes." If you have two "X" chromosomes as your 23rd pair, you are female. If mom gave you an "X" but dad gave you a "Y" type 23rd chromosome, you are genetically, male.

As crazy as it sounds, the system of AGCT is the same one in all living things on this planet. There is no other way. Does a tree look like a fruit fly or an Olympic sprinter? In terms of molecular biology, they are indistinguishable. Believe it or not, Hussein Bolt and a Bristlecone Pine both use the same universal code for their 22 amino acids.

When condensed prior to a cell's division into two daughters, chromosomes look like furry bowties, like two silk worms twisted together near the middle. The number of chromosomes in a eukaryotic nucleus can vary from just one in a jack jumper ant to over a thousand per nucleus in the adder's-tongue fern. Chickens and dogs possess 78 chromosomes in each nucleus whereas cabbage has only 18 chromosomes in the nucleus of each of its cells.

You might ask yourself, "How the heck does a cell keep track of which chromosomes go to which daughter?" Using humans as the example, each daughter cell needs 46 chromosomes. Each one gets one copy of chromosomes number 1 through 23, both the maternal and paternal versions. A daughter cell has no use for an extra 21st chromosome, endowing her with 47 but leaving her sister cell with only 45 chromosomes.

When the chromosomes are distributed unevenly in the egg (or in less than 10% of cases, the sperm) we can get a problem that is like having 53, not 52 cards in a deck. The most common viable form of this trisomy (or three sets of chromosome copies) is called Down's syndrome and it occurs usually because mom's egg had an extra copy of the 21st chromosome before joining with dad's 23, giving a grand total of 47 chromosomes per cell, not 46.

The answer to my earlier question of how dividing cells keep track of which chromosomes go to which daughter is currently "we don't know." What we do know is that before cell division, chromosomes line up like dancing partners at a Virginia Reel or a Soul Train if you will. Forty-six chromosomes, or chromosomes #1-23 from your mother and #1-23 from your father will go to daughter A on one side and a matching set of 46 will go to daughter B. Chromosomes destined for A and chromosomes destined for B line up opposite each other right before the cell divides.

The chromosomes are tethered to spider webs called microtubules at their midsection (the centromere) and also at the their ends (the telomeres) so when the cell splits right down the middle, half the dancers are pulled one way and the other half are pulled the other way. In this way, both daughters end up with perfect copies of 46 chromosomes: 23 from mom and 23 from dad.

This process happens billions of times a day in your body just as the same cell division dance is taking place in all cells of all plants and animals. As inefficient as it may seem, every eukaryotic cell carries with it the entire library of its genetic information. For humans, the sum total of our 46 chromosomes, listed as one long message, would roughly be the equivalent of 6 GB of information if you consider one A-T base pair to be a byte.

Stay with me because we're almost done with the bare necessities of genetic knowledge. Remember that one side of the zipper has the sense and the other has the anti-sense? Reading the DNA code in the sense direction would be like listening to The Beatles' song, "Revolution 9" normally. Anti-sense is like playing it backwards on a turntable with the hopes of making out some hidden message.

Each single strand of DNA has polarity like the positive and negative ends of a battery. One end of the DNA strand is known as the 5'end (read as "five prime") and the other is always the 3' end ("three prime"). It turns out that a DNA chain can only be assembled in one direction. I repeat: a DNA chain can only be assembled in one direction.

The sense strand that is assembled to match the anti-sense strand is called the leading strand because it is continuously and easily assembled in the 5' to 3' direction.

In contrast, assembling the anti-sense single strand that sits across from the sense single strand requires Okazaki fragments, which are discrete segments of 5' to 3' matching DNA that are 'backfilled' and connected like splicing a cassette tape hundreds of times as needed.

This unidirectional assembly is critical to understanding why telomeres must shorten every time one mother divides into two daughters. It is known as the "end replication problem" although I totally disagree with the pejorative term "problem." The "end replication problem," simply stated, is that you cannot assemble the anti-sense strand to the tip because the molecules doing the copying are not able to start exactly at the end. Therefore, every cell division results in the loss of 50 to 100 base pairs.

This failure to copy to the end results in what we call "replicative senescence" or aging from repeated copying of the DNA. It is as true as saying a ball can only bounce a percentage of the height that it is dropped from and has nothing to do with anything other than simple mechanics.

"Every dogma has its day"
— Anthony Burgess

Here's an interesting question:

Q: Are cells immortal or do they a have limited number of divisions in them?

A: Yes!

Confused? Well the answer is both. Or rather, it depends on how 'stem-like' they are and how much telomerase activity they possess. I am not a big fan of dichotomy: good versus evil, Democrat versus Republican, etc. But in the case of whether cells are immortal or not, two opposing scientists embody this debate nicely: Alexis Carrel and Leonard Hayflick.

Alexis Carrel, representing cellular immortality, claimed to keep cells from a chicken heart alive for over 20 years from 1912 to 1932. Sound incredible? Well, there is a cell line from a woman named Henrietta Lacks called HeLA that represents her cervical cancer cells and they are still used for standardized lab testing today because they are still alive and reproducing. Read more in Rebecca Skloot's bestseller, *The Immortal Life of Henrietta Lacks* (Broadway Books, 2011). Incidentally, TA-65, a telomerase-activator mentioned later in this book, was validated as being a telomerase activator on Henrietta's immortal cervical cells.

In the "cells are not immortal" camp is Leonard Hayflick who put differentiated skin cells into a dish and found they became non-viable and dysfunctional within 40-50 cellular divisions or doublings. This beloved "Hayflick Limit" is in keeping with many people's limiting beliefs about our own potential immortality.

We will discuss it further in Chapter 5: "Stem Cells," but trust me when I tell you that there are two generally recognized traits of "stemness." First, is the ability to self-immortalize (which is directly correlated to telomerase activity, described in the next chapter). The second trait of stemness is the ability to divide asymmetrically. Asymmetric division means that a mother stem cell is capable of dividing into two distinct types of daughter cells: an identical mother stem cell copy and a more committed and differentiated daughter cell.

Carrel's embryonic cells were sufficiently undifferentiated enough "mother stem cells" types so they were self-immortalizing. In contrast, Hayflick's cells were telomerase-inactive daughter cells, destined to "burn out" like all non-stem/non-telomerase-active cell types.

So now we see that both Alexis Carrell and Leonard Hayflick were right. It's just that they were constrained by a false dichotomy!

So, What is a Telomere?

We can now understand why telomeres exist, or at least what "purpose" they appear to serve. This is related to what happens to the cells' chromosomes when their telomeres get too short, or the fuses burn down to the firecracker. This understanding was elucidated by Hermann Muller, a research scientist in Woods' Hole in the 1930s, twenty years before Watson and Crick described the DNA's double helical structure.

Muller's experiments involved irradiating fruit flies to produce mutants with deletions and inversions involving the ends of chromosomes. High energy rays produce DNA breaks, which is why UV exposure promotes skin cancer. Although Muller's DNA damage was artificially generated, the same uncapping is inevitable in telomeres as they erode from the replicative senescence that we just learned about.

"Of note, he never found mutants with deletions or inversions involving the natural ends of the chromosomes and concluded that: 'the terminal gene must have a special function, that of **sealing the end of the chromosome,** *so to speak, and that for*

some reason a chromosome cannot persist indefinitely without having its ends thus sealed.'

Muller coined the term telomere for this terminal gene from the Greek, meaning simply "end part," but the fact that this region of the chromosome deserved a specific name was a recognition that something unusual was going on there."

–Excerpted from: McKnights article,
  "Plant Telomere Biology", *The Plant Cell, April 2004*

Muller used experiment and observation to correctly deduce the function of telomeres long before we even knew the structure of DNA. In short, telomeres cap and protect the ends of the DNA like the plastic tips of shoelaces.

Teleologically (no pun intended), the reason DNA can't exist uncapped is due to a critical process, always on, known as "double-strand breakage repair." When the enzymes responsible for genetic surveillance "see" an uncapped chromosome end, it "thinks" that the cut end needs to be rejoined to another cut end. To the double-strand breakage repair "team" inside the nucleus, it's as if Hermann Muller made one clean ultraviolet zap to slice a chromosome and the team needs to tape those ends back together again.

Now we can view the system with a clear understanding based in function, biochemistry, and that is sound from an evolutionary standpoint. Uncapped ends of DNA (or ones with critically-short telomeres from replicative senescence) are recognized by the double-strand breakage repair mechanisms and then inappropriately attached or spliced to existing, capped chromosomes.

When one chromosome is attached to another, we get double chromosomes, like two trapeze artists Krazy Glued at the hands. The next time the mutant double chromosome or double trapeze artist is pulled apart, they will tear not at the hands, but at the shoulders or somewhere else, leading to endless possibilities of mutation.

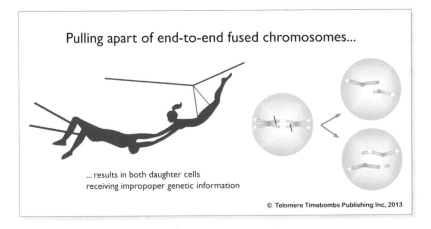

Pulling apart of end-to-end fused chromosomes...

... results in both daughter cells receiving impropoper genetic information

© Telomere Timebombs Publishing Inc, 2013

Fused chromosomes will result in uneven distribution to daughter cells

Because of double-strand breakage repair, telomere shortening leads to double chromosomes, which leads to uneven segregation and that process cannot be corrected but rather worsens with each cell division. This is not a "bad" thing. It is a part of the system that is expected and dealt with by many mechanisms. It is only when the master copy stem cells acquire errors and fail to self-destruct that we encounter problems.

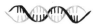

"This Tape Will Self-destruct in Five Seconds..."

The final tool we need for complete understanding of my stem cell theory of aging is called "apoptosis" or the unfortunately named "programmed cell death." Since DNA erosion at the telomeres is inevitable, the splicing and mutation of the genome (a term describing the sum total of a cell's chromosomes) is also inevitable. When the chromosomes line up to divide, if there is an asymmetry detected by what's called the "spindle assembly checkpoint," the cell's division can be prevented, effectively preventing mutation to propagate to the next generation of daughters.

Spindle assembly checkpoint activation is like a fire alarm. It indicates the chromosomal pairing is not symmetric, or that one player will get 51 cards and the other will be getting 53. The activated checkpoint signals the enzyme p53, which is known as the "watchman of the genome" because of its central role in recognizing and responding to genetic damage.

When p53 decides it is time to activate the apoptosis or death program, it signals that cell's battery acid-containing mitochondria to melt the host cell like the Wicked Witch of the East taking a shower. This is accomplished by essentially poking holes in the cell's thousands of mitochondria, which are filled with a sort of battery acid.

This purposeful melting from within explains the red herring of mitochondrial damage and oxidation seen in older cells. I believe those features are not the cause of aging as most people currently believe, but rather the result of the damaged cell's attempt to self-destruct.

This "oxidation as a red herring" hypothesis will not sit well with many people who are deeply invested in their theories of aging and pushing anti-oxidants, but in my opinion, it is hard-to-vary and therefore a better explanation.

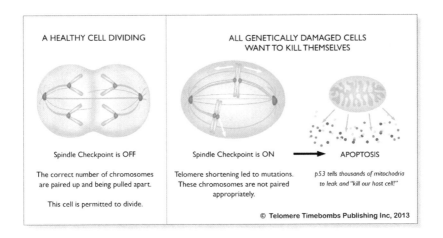

Damaged cells want to kill themselves by apoptosis

We must understand that apoptosis is a key function of every cell. In a variety of ways, cells are constantly checking for their own defects and willing and able to kill themselves if and when their own genetic damage is severe enough.

In the case of differentiated cells, like those that Leonard Hayflick studied, this is a good thing. As a thought experiment, if all cells were immortal and dividing, then within hours we would all become giant unsustainable blobs because two immortal cells would become 4, 8, 16, 32, etc., geometrically expanding into infinity and beyond, to borrow a phrase.

In the case of less differentiated, more stem-like cells like the ones that Carrel kept alive for 20 years, apoptosis was not widespread because the telomere fuses were maintained in length by telomerase. This prevents the inevitable telomere shortening, inappropriate splicing, mutation by uneven segregation at cell division, p53 activation, and mitochondrially-mediated self-destruction from ever taking place.

Did you know that chemotherapy works by the same mechanism? The goal of chemotherapy is to cause a lot of genetic damage in rapidly-reproducing cells so that the innate error detection mechanisms will kick in and apoptosis can occur. However, DNA mutation will eventually lead to more cancers down the road so a more precisely directed solution is desirable.

Causing DNA damage with chemotherapy to cure cancer is kind of like trying to solve inner city gang violence by sending in more guns and removing teachers and police officers.

In conclusion, chromosomes are simply long, paired DNA strands that contain instructions for RNA messages that are subsequently translated into proteins. Erosion is inevitable because of mechanical reasons and that is a good thing except in stem cells.

When the telomeres erode too much, stem the cell's repair mechanisms initiate new splices that will spell the doom for future descendants because chromosomal mutation from uneven separation at cell division will trigger p53 to cause apoptosis or cell suicide.

Twenty years in a dish? Just how did those chicken heart stem cells manage that? That is the subject of our next chapter describing a magical, mystical enzyme called telomerase.

4

TELOMERASE

"Humans were so stupid. They had something so precious, and they barely safeguarded it at all. They threw away their lives for money, for packets of powder, for a stranger's charming smile."

— Cassandra Clare, <u>City of Bones</u>
(Margaret K. McElderry Books, 2008)

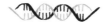

Take a deep breath and exhale. Repeat as necessary. Congratulations! If you have made it to this point in the book, you have acquired all the information that you will need to understand why we age, how it can be prevented, and understand more than 99.999% of the medical doctors that you will meet at the time of this writing. You could rightly consider yourself a bit of genius, in my opinion.

This chapter is about telomerase and its role in maintaining telomeres in the stem cells of your body. The chapter after this one will explore stem cells.

Think of telomerase as a stock ticker tape machine, or for those younger than the baby boom generation, like those Acco adhesive label makers that you perhaps used to label your school locker, or for those even younger, a Brother P-Touch label maker.

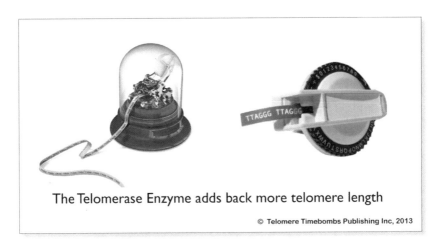

The Telomerase Enzyme adds back more telomere length

© Telomere Timebombs Publishing Inc, 2013

Telomerase can keep stem cells young

The primary role of the telomerase enzyme is to add more telomere to the ends of chromosomes, thereby lengthening those fuses and adding time to your cells' lifespans.

So this chapter is really about hope. Telomerase rescues cells, and therefore couldn't it rescue us from aging and dying? Or perhaps there is some ironic, unintended come-uppance, such as cancer, that will result from harnessing the power of this immortalizing enzyme?

Now it's time to tell you that telomere caps are not special molecules per se. They are also comprised of DNA, folded back on itself exactly like a paper clip. Our human telomeres consist of a six base pair sequence that reads GGGATT in the 5' to 3' sense direction, repeated over and over. In plants, the message is 7 base pairs. In some fungi, the message is 23 base pairs repeated. The fact that the evolution of eukaryotes has conserved the function of telomeres while allowing exact telomere "text" to change, implies the critical importance of having some kind of blank tape message at the ends of your DNA.

In 1953, Watson and Crick, 20 years after Muller correctly inferred the role of telomeres as protective caps, won the Nobel Prize in medicine for describing the exact structure of DNA as a continuous strand of those four molecules of DNA (AGC&T) mated to a complementary strand, which are both coiled up into a double helix.

In 2009, three scientists won the Nobel Prize in medicine and physiology for having described the role of telomerase. This is the exact wording of the Nobel Panel: "The Nobel Prize in Physiology or Medicine 2009 was awarded jointly to Elizabeth H. Blackburn, Carol W. Greider and Jack W. Szostak *"for the discovery of how chromosomes are protected by telomeres and the enzyme telomerase"*.

And just how does telomerase do this? First of all, let's describe what telomerase truly is. Telomerase is a micromachine assembled from several proteins and it works primarily in the cell's nucleus to constantly repair the shortening ends by adding back length. I don't know how many telomerase molecules are at work simultaneously, but it is not just one, but many.

The telomerase enzyme complex, human telomere reverse transcriptase (or hTERT for short) can attach to a stem cell's telomeres at each of the ninety-six 5' to 3' leading strands. It prefers to lengthen short ones and there is a mechanism for pruning so they don't get excessively long.

Telomerase actively writes or adds back more length in a process known as reverse transcription. Briefly, it is called "reverse" because it flips the central dogma of genetics, namely that DNA is translated into RNA. Thus, telomerase engages in this reverse process: using an RNA template to produce DNA. When you think about it, because human telomere reads GGGTTA from 5' to 3', our RNA matching complimentary template would read CCCUUT from 3' to 5' (U is for Uracil, the RNA chains' particular flavor of (A)denosine).

This telomerase RNA template (hereafter referred to as TERC) is like a key that is needed to run the telomerase engine. This TERC key combines with a molecule called dyskerin, that stabilizes it. Together, the TERC/dyskerin pair are needed to allow telomerase hTERT to attach and properly lengthen the overhanging 3' leading strand. Remember DNA can only be made in the 5' to 3' direction.

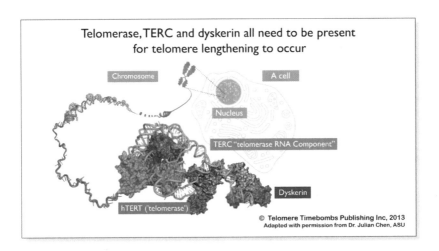

**A TERC+dyskerin "key" is needed
for the telomerase engine to work**

So if all cells have the hTERT, the TERC "key", and the dyskerin, why don't all cells lengthen their telomeres?

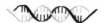

Telomerase production is turned off in non-stem cells

In humans, telomerase production is retained in the immortal stem cells. With increasing cellular differentiation, telomerase production is turned off using epigenetic modifications, possibly at the promoter region upstream from the hTERT gene. Telomerase activity may also be turned off and on by other pathways and by post-transcriptional modifications to the TERC "key".

What happens if the telomerase-mediated reverse transcription isn't working well in our stem cells? Nature has done that experiment and the answer is an accelerated aging syndrome known as progeria, which is the direct result of abnormal TERC/dyskerin function. More on this in Chapter 7: "Aging slow, fast, and not at all."

One important fact that isn't intuitively obvious to most people is that the telomerase enzymes are assembled for use in only that cell, indeed in that nucleus. Telomerase is not something that floats around like glucose, free to travel around the blood stream to all cells. That is why you can't simply ingest a telomerase pill. It would be destroyed by your stomach acid just like every other complex protein is quickly broken down by digestion.

So what happens when an abnormally large number of copies of telomerase are available after ingesting a telomerase *activator*?

This will be explored in Chapter 9: "Telomerase activation medicine" but in a nutshell, the normal reparative and restorative functions of telomerase are enhanced, thereby producing a reversal of the changes associated with aging.

The wonderful thing about science is that you reduce scale to deduce causation and observe and test those theories. But a reductionist approach has difficulty explaining the more complex interactions emerging from the individual biochemical pathways. Suffice it to say that telomeres do not overextend, as there is a trimming mechanism. If that were not the case, my telomeres wouldn't have stopped lengthening just under 10,000 base pairs after 6 years of ingesting a telomerase activator. Incidentally, at the age of 46, my telomeres measure out to be like those of a teenager now!

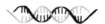

What does Telomere Measurement Really Tell Us?
Now is a good time to discuss telomere length. Telomere length is how many base pairs a chromosome has on its tip. This length is inherited from the mother cell that made the daughter. There is no great mystery in this because the process of copying DNA in the six base pair repeating end is the same as in the more central regions of the chromosome.

When an egg is fertilized, the length of the single cell's telomeres are reset, like a pinball machine would reset to a score of zero when starting a new game. That original length is generally around 15,000 base pairs for a human. By the time the baby is born, it has already burned through a third of his life expectancy and has only 10,000 base pairs remaining. This is because the telomerase activity is inadequate to sustain the 15,000 base pair length in the presence of the rapid cell copying that is required to produce a baby from a single egg in thirty-eight weeks of pregnancy.

All cells can be only as good or as young as their mother. I repeat: all cells can be only as good or as young as their mother. When I say "good," I mean the integrity of the genetic message. When I say "young" I mean the inherited length of the telomeres. There are other so-called epigenetic changes that are also important in determining cell age. But for the most part, the age of a cell is a function of the inevitable result of the "end replication problem" and the replicative senescence that we discussed in Chapter 3: "What is a telomere?"

It is worth it to try to understand whether each cell, prior to division, has 184 telomeres or 368. The cell spends most of its time with only a single copy of its chromosomes because it is not planning to split just yet. That means it has 23 chromosomes from mom and 23 from dad. A good way to remember this is that the 23rd chromosome is either an X from mom or an X or Y from dad. But the other 22 chromosomes also have a maternal and paternal versions.

Prior to cell division, a full library of 92 chromosomes is prepared: 46 for each of the two post-division daughters. Every chromosome is comprised of a pair of strands with two tips on each end. They read GGGATT 5' to 3' and CCCTAA in the 3' to 5' direction, up to a 15,000 base pairs in length. So, 4 x 92 = 368.

On the other hand, you could also argue that there are 184 telomeres because the 5' and 3' ends spend most of their time combined in what is called "shelterin," or the paperclip-like tip of the tip. Both strands and the rest of the shelterin complex form a single functional unit of a telomere.

The reason I bothered to explain about individual chromosomes is that the concept of someone's "telomere length" is often, in fact almost always, misunderstood as a single number. After the Nobel Prize in 2009, an idiotic although engaging news tagline was making the rounds. It asked, "If there was a test to tell you when you would die, would you take it? Well now there is! Tune in, to this evening's news...."

The life expectancy test they were referring to is called the leukocyte telomere length (LTL) measurement. It is a calculation of the median length of chromosomal telomeres in the white blood cells (also known as leukocytes). But telomere erosion doesn't occur in a predictable fashion. When we examine the predicted lengths for a 10-year-old or a 100-year-old, the 95% confidence intervals, or the values encompassing 95% of the people in that age group, overlap almost completely. In other words, you can't predict a person's age from their median telomere length with any accuracy. In addition, measuring the LTL won't necessarily tell you about what's happening throughout the body. We check leukocyte telomere length because it's easy to draw blood but its value is dubious when it comes to predicting anything, let alone the day of your demise.

Another reason why a telomere length measurement does not predict the length of your life is really quite simple. Every cell has up to 184 telomeres in its nucleus that can and in fact do, vary quite a bit in their individual lengths. Above a certain length, let us say 2500 base pairs, there is little danger of the kind of re-splicing mutation by the "double-strand breakage team" that is ever-vigilant.

It only takes a single one of those 184 telomeres to be naked or uncapped in an immortal stem cell in order to start the progressive "confettization" of your pristine genetic endowment. Absent an accidental trauma, the date of your demise will depend upon available medical care and many coexisting potential diseases in many organ systems, which are themselves comprised of many stem cell niches, that are themselves dependent on their stem cells' ability to recognize their damage and self-annihilate (undergo apoptosis), and also their ability to be replaced by better, more functional stem cells. This does not include the immune system, the extracellular (outside the cells) matrices and the micro-nutritional, microbial, and toxic milieu in which those cells operate. Sorry for the run-on sentence before-- it is intended to illustrate the absurdity of that news teaser.

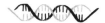

A Parable to Illustrate the Absurdity of Using LTL to Predict Anything

There is always a danger in anthropomorphizing (thinking of things in human terms) but here is a hard-working analogy that would illustrate why that news teaser was so absurd. That news premise would be like saying the date of the end of the Vietnam War was decided by the hair on the soldiers' heads in one skirmish. Let's explore.

Pretend telomere length is hair length and cells are the soldiers. It is 1972 and let us say that creeping in some foxhole a year from now, on the other side of the planet, a young Vietnamese soldier will decide whether to shoot you from behind based on whether he sees the same red birthmark that his younger brother has, at the base of your neck, just above the hairline.

On the day you show up to Parris Island for boot camp you may have long, hippie-like hair after returning from a summer in San Francisco. On the first day, it's clear that average hair length wouldn't tell you much about where any Marine recruit came from, what his religious background or vocational endowment was, or most importantly whether he will ask for the shorter or longer clipper attachment during his final leave before possibly being ambushed. It wouldn't tell you which platoon he was assigned to, which patrol, how good his hearing was. But somehow we can predict the future based on what?

Stop everything. Soldiers put down your guns. American GIs and Viet Cong take off your helmets. Everyone shave your head bald. Each soldier, hand me in a plastic bag with the hair from the 4 cm^2 above your right ear (not even where your birthmark would be). From measuring the average weight of hair, how could I possibly tell you whether or not Cpl. Nguyen sees the birthmark and the humanity in Cpl. Browning, spares his life, and creeps silently back into the jungle?

How can knowing average hair length predict the end of the war? If you can explain that then I will accept that LTL can predict the date of your death.

I have just touched upon the dirty little secret of the massive field of telomere research. The presumption that a person's median LTL is correlated with other disease conditions is held as axiomatic, but it is counterintuitive, baseless, and supremely EASY-to-vary. We should be wary of drawing conclusions from just that one measurement. We will explore this further in Chapter 6: "Telomere erosion in disease."

Having said that, leukocyte telomere measurements are something that I routinely use, absolutely endorse and believe in, and something that I believe can provide a valuable benchmark for telomerase activation therapy.

How can I reconcile my apparent disdain for telomere measurements and my complete faith in them? It is because telomere dysfunction leading to stem cell dysfunction, leading to disease and organ dysfunction, takes place right there in the barbershop in Da Nang. It is literally just one minor detail, or critically-short telomere that will determine the cell's fate. It is not the average length of hair on that soldier's scalp, the way the platoon wears its hair, or who is in the White House that matters. This is a time when anthropomorphisms are appropriate.

New analogy. It is easy to check tire tread. But can we use tire tread wear to predict how the brakes, carburetor, or headlamps are performing? Behind that presumption is that wear takes place equally among all parts of the car in an evenly distributed manner and is not subject to temporal or regional variation, and cannot be in a state of constant maintenance and repair. That is the presumption we are making when naively attempt to correlate white blood cell telomere length with other disease conditions.

In conclusion, telomerase is always active but only functions properly in our immortalized stem cells. Telomerase enzymes are constantly trying to preserve, protect, and even destroy host stem cells through the body. In my opinion, we must be cautious about using median telomere length as anything more than a benchmark for telomerase activation therapy.

As we will discuss in the next chapter, disease is a property that emerges from stem cell dysfunction, which can be decided by the shortening of one single telomere. And that, my friends, is why it is important to keep your telomere fuses from eroding in the first place.

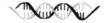

5

STEM CELLS

*"[The altruist's act of suicide] springs from hope;
for it depends on the belief in beautiful perspectives
beyond this life."*
— From *Suicide*, by Sociologist Emile Durkheim

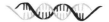

In recent years, the idea of extracting stem cells and reintroducing them into a patient for therapy has become more accepted. What probably never should have happened was the infusion of xenograft stem cells, meaning stem cells which come from non-human species. That is because non-human cells are rapidly destroyed by our immune systems, which recognize them as hostile. Also questionable is the industry of stem cell tourism that falsely promises miracle cures to people.

There are, as a matter of knee-jerk response, many people who consider what I do in activating telomerase as a similar kind of cynical opportunism. But as we will discuss in Chapter 9: "Telomerase activation medicine," the scientific basis is sound and the anecdotes are very consistent and compelling.

So ask yourself, would it be safer and more cost effective to extract, process, and reintroduce your own stem cells, or fix the stem cells that already exist, right where they live, by ingesting a safe capsule derived from an herb? That is precisely what I believe telomerase activation medicine does.

And if you could, would you rather prevent damage to your stem cells or destroy and replace damaged ones? As we'll see in this chapter, both of these processes are always at work to ward off aging and disease.

In this chapter, we will learn five essential things that form the basis of stem cell biology:

1) To explain how cell differentiation is like the game Stratego™;

2) Explain why changes to the DNA, called epigenetic modifications, are like the software in a generic personal computer;

3) Convince you that cancer is a stem cell disease just as Clark Kent and not Jimmy Olsen is Superman;

4) Show that stem cells are like queen bees in their hives; and

5) Explain how a special type of stem cell, the mesenchymal stem cell, is like a frozen food that can be thawed and served when you need new stem cells.

Just to recap, "stemness" is defined by two traits: self-immortalization (due to telomerase activity) and asymmetric division (making a perfect clone of itself as a mother stem cell and a more differentiated daughter when it divides). There are specific markers that can be used to practically identify them but let's keep in mind that "stemness" is a bit vague and abstract, like truth and beauty.

Even more problematic is that the behavior of stem cells is still a mystery. I like to think of "stemness" as being on a continuum, like that old board game, Stratego.

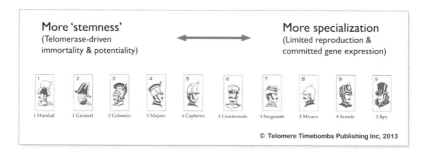

Cell differentiation is kind of like Stratego

In the game, there are a few powerful pieces but more of the weaker pieces. The weakest of the pieces have highly specific functions, such as scouting or defusing bombs. If cell potentiality is like Stratego combat ability, then the zygote (or fertilized egg) would be like the all-powerful Marshal piece, because it is better than all the rest and has the potential to become all types of cells.

After the single zygote, subsequent generations of cells lose stemness and potentiality in exchange for specialization. Mixing analogies, as they commit to certain types of cell lines and organs the Marshal becomes a General, two Colonels, four Lieutenants and eight Scouts. For example, a skin stem cell's ancestors started out from the fertilized egg, then they became stem cells known as ectodermal, then through stepwise differentiation achieved through epigenetic switches of a sort, they eventually became committed to making copies of themselves and skin cells.

Programming or stem cell damage can cause terminal differentiation to occur. This terminal or final differentiation means they lose their stemness, and no longer make an immortal mother and mortal sister-daughter. Once dedicated to a more specific lineage, cells usually don't go backwards and dedifferentiate.

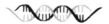

Epigenetic Changes are the Software of the Cell

If you're still following me then I was right about one thing, you are a genius! Now, let us introduce a very important concept known as epigenetics. This is the study of how modifications to the chromosomes, often near to some key genes determining cell differentiation, are added in order to alter the functioning of that cell. Think of each cell as a huge library that has only one or two large tables that can be covered with open books to read. The majority of the books are unread, just like the majority of the genes are coiled up and hidden away from actually expression or translation into proteins.

Before epigenetics, scientists seemed to think that DNA sequences alone somehow explained cell behavior, although there wasn't a great theoretical framework to explain how that would work. Now, we are beginning to understand that what's essential isn't just having the genes, because all the cells possess all genes, it is the manner in which they are expressed that is at the heart of determining a cell's function and path of differentiation. I mean, how could you get anything done if all 6 gigabytes of library text were all splayed out on the tables, chairs and floor of your library? These epigenetic changes dictate whether cells will act like Stratego lieutenants or miners, shall we say. That is the key to how our cell differentiation system works.

Think of cells and their fully loaded 6 gigabytes of DNA as computer hardware, like a generic, no-name personal computer. The epigenetic modifications comprise the operating system and software applications and will dictate how the cell communicates as well as how it functions.

Epigenetic changes are primarily determined by purposeful chemical additions to the DNA known as acetylation (adding an acetyl group) and methylation (adding a methyl group) or by the use of specialized types of attached RNA (a slightly different version of DNA). It is critical to understand that it is not only the DNA library that is copied for both daughters, but also the mother cell's epigenetic modifications. That makes sense otherwise a liver cell would be able to make bone cells, which it generally doesn't do. It would be cumbersome and inefficient to have to recreate every step of differentiation from a Marshall zygote to a Corporal, and much easier to start with the epigenetic marks that mom already has.

Analogy downshift: In medieval times, your name was Miller or Baker because your ancestors were literally millers or bakers. You didn't need your kids to go to school to learn any other trades; they picked up the family business.

Now that you understand these concepts, I have a bonus question for you: would the epigenetic changes of a stem cell be symmetric prior to dividing? Probably not! The more differentiated daughter would have slightly altered, more differentiated sets of epigenetic marks compared to its mother and its sister/mother for the next generation. Remember, asymmetric division was one of the two qualities of stemness.

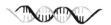

Cancer is Mainly a Disease of Stem Cells

The other trait of stemness is immortality due to telomerase activation. Most cancers have high telomerase activity leading many, even Nobel Prize winners, to speculate that taking telomerase activators might create or allow cancer in me and other folks taking TA-65. Tens of thousands of people have ingested the telomerase activator since 2005, and cancer rates do not appear to have increased in us. Why not?

There is a new orthodoxy emerging known as the "cancer stem cell" theory. It holds that the reason telomerase activity is present in cancers is because it is retained, not reactivated. In other words, cancers don't originate in telomerase-inactive differentiated cells but rather from already telomerase-active stem cells.

There is, in fact, growing evidence that because a large tumor may be replenished by these Marshall-like super-powered cancer stem cells, if we can find and kill those special cancer stem cells, the remainder of the malignant cells might just burn themselves out via replicative senescence.

When I was in medical school in 1989, they taught us that cancer happened when ordinary cells achieved a few specific mutations that would allow for uncontrolled growth, movement, and replication. In my opinion, this was scientific dogma based on received wisdom rather than careful thought or evidence.

Think for a moment. If you wanted to create a deadly cancer, would you choose Carrell's chicken embryos or Hayflick's damaged old skin cells? How hard would it be to take a damaged cell and further damage it into a stable, mutated and de-differentiated stem cell? Wouldn't you choose a cell that was already immortal, then slightly tweak that robust and otherwise hale and hearty cell?

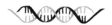

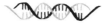

Parable Illustrating Why Cancer is Probably from Stem Cells Gone Bad

Imagine a hundred people standing around while a piano falls from the sky onto a Boy Scout troop. If your name is Jimmy Olsen, you might get a great photo, but unless your name is Clark Kent you won't be able to do much about it.

Because Clark was born on the Planet Krypton, the rules of strength and gravity on Earth don't apply to him in the same way. Same with stem cells. They are already superheroes of a sort, self-immortalizing with telomerase, and much more genetically pristine than a run-of-the-mill citizen of Metropolis.

If a stem cell stops playing nice with its neighbors (what we refer to in cell biology as loss of contact inhibition), or travels where it doesn't belong (metastasis) then we have a super villain, like a "Bizarro Superman". In most cases, it would be harder to get an old and damaged, already differentiated cell to de-differentiate and somehow activate its telomerase, but that doesn't mean it can't and doesn't happen. It's just not the easier and more logical way to achieve clinical malignancy.

A nice aspect to this stem cell theory of cancer is that we might only have to target a few cells to cure cancer because most tumors are monoclonal. That means they are all genetically identical because they are derived from one single mutated cancer stem cell. If we could find and kill that one bad cell, the others could eventually burn out.

Analogy downshift: if you wanted to survive the grizzly reptilo-insectoid monsters of the *Alien* movies, would you go after the little horseshoe crab-like critters or try to torch the egg-laying mother?

How is a Stem Cell like a Queen Bee?

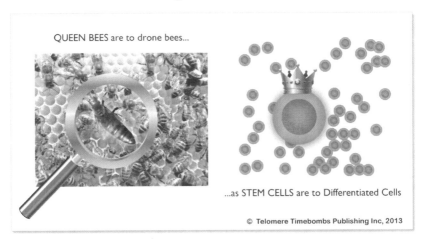

QUEEN BEES are to drone bees...

...as STEM CELLS are to Differentiated Cells

© Telomere Timebombs Publishing Inc, 2013

Stem cells are like queen bees

Like the big bad mama alien, queen bees live many years and can reproduce themselves nearly infinitely. In contrast, drone bees are mere clones of the mother and live only months at best. This is a great analogy for stem cells because they too are immortal whereas their differentiated daughter clones are destined to burn out after forty divisions (perhaps a few months) due to replicative senescence.

The analogy can be extended because there is one queen per hive and likewise, there is probably just one stem cell per niche. A niche is a finite area of cells surrounding a stem cell that are all genetically identical because they are all derived from that one cell.

To illustrate the concept of niches, let's say an organ like the liver has 100 stem cell niches like a beekeeper has 100 hives.

If the liver is exposed to global poisoning, like chronic viral infection or alcohol exposure, all the queens will be damaged and all the drones will be damaged according to the same general trends. But the precise mutations will vary in each niche despite the assumption and gross outward appearance of a field-like phenomenon being applied equally. Remember, the daughters can only be as healthy (good genetic integrity) or as young (telomere length) as their stem cell mother and each niche has a different mother.

This means that liver cancer doesn't happen in all 100 niches gradually. It usually strikes in only one niche and spreads. That is what most cancerous organs demonstrate at autopsy. We know the tumor cells have a monoclonal origin because they all possess the same exact DNA damage signature, if you will. But the 99 other niches and their queens and drones possess mutations unlike the currently cancerous one. This makes sense and when studied by genetic analysis, is demonstrated to be true. And we love it when those things occur together because they are what? That's right: hard-to-vary.

In comparing good organ health with organ dysfunction we are reminded of that wonderful opening line of *Anna Karenina*: "All happy families are happy in the exact same way. All unhappy families are unhappy in their own unique fashion." Just so with a happy, young liver. All niches are filled with original factory liver cells. With damage, all of the liver cells accumulate their unique mutations and eventually, given enough time, many will become cancerous as a result of a single queen bee stem cell gone awry, not the de-differentiation of her damaged and short-lived drones.

So a TV Dinner Could Save my Life?

The final goal of this chapter was to explain about frozen food, right? Well it turns out that when you kill the queen bee, a drone is fed royal jelly and becomes a queen. Interestingly, this is where the analogy breaks down. In your body, when a queen-like stem cell becomes genetically damaged and the p53 pokes holes in the mitochondria to initiate apoptosis, promotion doesn't come from within, but from without.

There is a special type of itinerant less differentiated queen-like stem cell that is constantly circulating and looking for such an abdicated throne. It is called a "mesenchymal stem cell." Although mesenchymal implies that it only makes specific types of cells, in fact, it probably can become nearly any type of required stem cell.

These mesenchymal stem cells are thought to be preserved in our cartilage, like a *Jurassic Park* (Universal Pictures, 1993) insect trapped in amber millions of years ago. Maybe a better analogy would be like having stacks of Hungry Man® sirloin steak dinners that you stored away in 1976. Really, this is quite an elegant design because as non-dividing and inactive cells, they were frozen in time and their genetic integrity is that of a young child, or at least not so old and damaged as the person that you might be at this time.

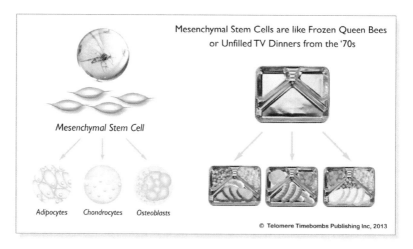

Mesenchymal Stem Cells are like Frozen Queen Bees or Unfilled TV Dinners from the '70s

Mesenchymal Stem Cell

Adipocytes   Chondrocytes   Osteoblasts

© Telomere Timebombs Publishing Inc, 2013

Mesenchymal stem cells can be "defrosted" into different types

With many current stem cell infusion therapies, stem cells are overloaded into the system. While it may provide some benefits, that method ignores the root cause of the problem. The stem cell queens that currently occupying their niches' thrones aren't stepping down and killing themselves, even though there are millions of would-be mesenchymal stem cells that could replace them.

Analogy downshift: if we go back to our liver with 100 queendoms or niches and think of them as chairs in a high school auditorium, we can't get more than 100 people seated in that auditorium (even if we stacked chairs on top of other chairs). There are 100 old people parked in those seats, and thousands of young people waiting outside to get in.

Mixing analogies, we need to encourage those damaged, older people to "take one for the team" and kill themselves. One by one, a damaged Queen, in her honeycomb or niche, is replaced by a mesenchymal stem cell that was waiting outside the auditorium for just that opportunity. And that, my friends, is the essence of how we are designed to stay alive and healthy for as long as possible.

But rather than risk letting things get that bad, wouldn't it be better to prevent damage to those 100 queen bees before apoptosis and replacement by mesenchymal stem cells was needed? Of course! And just how we accomplish will be the subject of Chapter 7: "Aging slow, fast, and not at all."

To recap, we explained why cell differentiation is like the game Stratego, how epigenetics is like the software of the cells, why "Bizarro Superman" is at fault for cancer, we discussed why stem cells are Queen bees in their hives, and showed how the system replaces vacated thrones with younger, frozen versions.

This was a pretty meaty chapter with some pretty fast and furious analogy downshifting but hopefully you are starting to think, "Sounds plausible, Dr. Park, but what proof do you have if I don't want to go by your word alone?" I'm glad you asked, because that brings us to our next chapter.

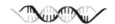

6

TELOMERE EROSION IN DISEASE

"When I see a bird that quacks like a duck, walks like a duck, has feathers and webbed feet and associates with ducks—I'm certainly going to assume that he IS a duck."

— Emil Mazey, Secretary-Treasurer,
United Automobile Workers

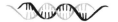

In this chapter, we will discuss only a few of the thousands of scientific articles linking the erosion of telomeres to the deterioration of health. The chapter following this one will specifically address the relationship of telomere erosion to the process of aging, which is a closely related topic.

In Chapter 1: "Why do we get old?" I explained why certain undisputed and obvious facts led me to imagine my stem cell theory of aging based upon telomere erosion. I compared current ignorance of the obvious basis of aging to the story of the "Emperor's New Clothes."

When I think about this plethora of hard, scientific evidence linking telomere erosion to all diseases, it reminds me of another naked monarch, the Lady Godiva, The Lady Godiva rode around the city streets, naked on a horse, while all but one Peeping Tom kept their shutters closed.

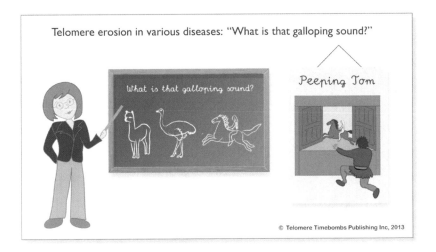

**Don't come up with many explanations
when a single one will suffice**

In labs across the world, science is showing a link between leukocyte telomere length and every disease condition. So why is each condition treated differently? Yes, I know I don't love the LTL as a proxy for aging in all organ systems, but hey, it's all we've got so we just roll with it.

Reductionist science assumes and asks us to believe that we are hearing zebras, griffins, donkeys and all manner of beasts trotting in the streets outside. I will play the role of the infamous Peeping Tom and ask you to cast open the shutters with me and gaze upon the Lady Godiva galloping around our city streets. That lady is telomere shortening and the horses are our various types of stem cells.

Even though you may not be a physician or scientist, by the end of this chapter you should be flabbergasted that telomere biology is not the central area of study for all diseases. Actually, it already is! However, it is as though there were 1,000 wheel factories feverishly trying to invent a wheel, when the high-speed automobile is already a reality.

We don't need another model. My telomere erosion/stem cell theory is hard-to-vary but we have a situation where scientists are making careers by proving a knife can cut through a carrot, and celery, and bread, etc. It's a knife! It can cut through a lot of things.

We simply don't need another study showing association between telomere damage and disease. We need randomized controlled trials with telomerase activators in a variety of disease conditions and we need them now.

I came up with a diagram consisting of concentric octagons that illustrates why I believe there is truly only one disease. Of course, diseases can also be brought about by trauma, infection, toxins, or inherited genetic anomalies, but the one disease of replicative senescence can account for most of what we experience as different disease conditions.

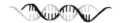

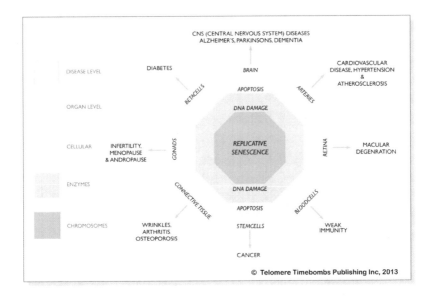

© Telomere Timebombs Publishing Inc, 2013

There is only one disease with many faces

In the innermost octagon, we encounter shortening of telomeres from replicative senescence, or the Lady Godiva riding all our horses.

The next octagon is the universal process of DNA damage that ironically comes from the DNA double-strand damage repair 'team' splicing uncapped telomeres into double chromosomes. This begets damage the next time the chromosomes line up for division because the chromosomes will be torn apart and distributed unevenly.

In the third octagon we have stem cell senescence and failed apoptosis of those stem cells. In other words, once the DNA of the immortal stem cells is damaged, they misbehave and display weird behaviors, acting crotchety like grumpy old men. This is not a problem unless the damage isn't severe enough to trigger apoptosis so that your "Snow White" mesenchymal stem cells can come and replace these old and Evil Queen bees.

In the fourth organ level octagon, we look at the various stem cell types that acquire damage. Different cells behave and also misbehave in distinct ways, which is why medical school takes four years and why there are so many wonderful research project opportunities.

The outermost manifestations of the one disease will depend upon the stem cell type that comprises the organ in question. For example, damage to neural stem cells of the brain will manifest as the diseases of Alzheimer's, Parkinson's, and even insomnia. Damage to stem cells of the heart and arteries manifests at the disease level as cardiovascular disease, hypertension, and stroke.

Damage to the blood-producing components will manifest as weakened immunity, anemia, and myelodysplasia (an age-related pre-leukemia).

Damage to pancreatic insulin-producing cells manifests as diabetes. From damage to the stem cells of the ovaries and testes, we get menopause and decreased testosterone and male sexual dysfunction. From damage to retinal stem cells, we manifest macular degeneration.

And so it goes, on and on until it begins to dawn on us that so many diseases increase in prevalence with age and that the overwhelming mountain of peer reviewed, scientific data support shortening of telomeres is associated with each and every one of these diseases.

David Deutsch would be pleased. This is an extremely "hard-to-vary" model and one that is unifying in its scope and simplicity.

Now let's get down to "brass tacks." This is an expression that I learned from my years of screenwriting, which comes from the brass tacks that you use to bind the pages of your script after having committed thoughts into words and paper.

We will briefly touch upon only a few highlights of this vast scientific literature that links telomere dysfunction with diabetes, hypertension, osteoporosis, arthritis, Alzheimer's, immune deficiency, and cancer. I encourage you to go to the National Institutes of Health website called "PubMed" where you can and should immediately type in any disease plus the word "telomere," to retrieve dozens to hundreds of citations.

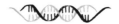

The "Rashomon" of Research

Rashomon (Daiei Motion Picture Company, 1950) was created by Japanese film director, Akira Kurosawa. It tells the story of a gentleman and his wife who encounter a brigand on the road. The brigand and the wife have sex and the husband is killed. Those are the facts. But the four retellings of the story, while not deviating from those facts, could not possibly be more different, illustrating the subjective nature of recollection, representation, and significance that is unavoidable in the human condition.

This leads us to a discussion about bias. We humans crave significance and meaning. We construct stories then reframe them, then abandon the original principles with which we began our journeys. That is the unavoidable truth of scientific, peer-reviewed research, observation, and life in a nutshell. We are embarrassed if our best laid plans of test tube mice and brilliant men come to naught. So, many scientists will consciously or subconsciously tweak, spin, and overreach in an attempt to reach significance, meaning, and gravitas in their work.

In research there are biases of study design, subject selection, non-random sampling, data collection, reporting, data interpretation, and interpretation to fit existing paradigms. The types of bias are endless so we should always salute the scientists who unabashedly report "I went looking for this thing, and didn't find it." Though it feels like failure, it really isn't. Reporting so-called negative results is as much a foundation of science as the absence of figure and form would be in a Matisse drawing, or the 60% failed at bats in baseball would contribute to a Hall of Fame 400 career batting average.

I have the utmost respect for researchers but we hope for "just the facts," as Sergeant Joe Friday of the TV show *Dragnet* would have it. If you take with a grain of salt the first and last sentences of each abstract (which is the one paragraph summary of the journey of the research project) then we have the meal. The first sentence is the restaurant review and the last is the group photo outside at the end of the meal. The proof of the pudding is in the eating and so it is food or facts presented in every study that we must consume and digest on our own.

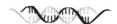

Hair Graying, Nail Growth, and Wrinkles

When cells undergo replicative senescence, the DNA is damaged. When this occurs in keratin-producing stem cells, we get the hallmarks of old age, both in "normal" people and people with only half a gene dose of telomerase, or progeria-affected children.

Those manifestations are loss of and graying of the hair, poor nail growth, and wrinkling of the skin.

Siegl-Cachedenier et al, in the *Journal of Cell Biology* (2007), showed that when telomerase was increased in aging mice, their hair follicle stem cells improved in their ability to move and reproduce and there were fewer critically-shortened telomeres associated with them as well. The hair grew better, the mice lived longer, and there was no increased cancer incidence.

As we will discuss in Chapter 9 "Telomerase activation medicine," better growth of hair, skin and nails is documented in mice after telomerase activation. Anecdotally, I also have seen hair repigmentation, even in patients over 110 years old!

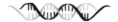

Diabetes is Aging of the Pancreatic Beta Cells

Maria Blasco, the director of the Spanish National Cancer Institute, is the preeminent researcher in telomere and telomerase science in my opinion. She worked in the Cold Springs Harbor lab of Carol Greider, one of the Nobel Prize winners for the discovery of telomerase.

Blasco's laboratory gave TA-65 (a telomerase activator) to mice engineered to age rapidly by knocking out one copy of their TERC gene. Recall from Chapter 4: "Telomerase" that a correct TERC/dyskerin RNA "key" is needed for the telomerase "engine" to access the chromosome's 3' end and lengthen the telomere. She found that their glucose tolerance improved after TA as did their osteoporosis and skin health (see Bernardes de Jesus et al in *The Aging Cell* (2011). Anecdotally, I have seen this in many of my patients as well. A randomized controlled trial to evaluate whether TA affects glucose tolerance could be done quickly and cost-effectively.

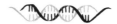

High Blood Pressure is the Cure, not the Disease

The walls of the arteries are made of smooth lining, like Teflon®, that coats the inside tube, or what we call the lumen. Artery walls contain muscles to contract and propel blood forward and they have elastin, a stretchy rubber-like substance that allows the artery to expand a bit and store the energy from pumping that will be released when the system is resting. The *Windkessel Effect* ('wind chamber,' in German) is the description of just that. It's like squeezing a balloon animal; the distension and stretching of the elastin stores energy that will be released in a healthy artery.

As the arteries age, elastin is lost, and the artery can bulge. This typically happens in the main outflow of the heart called the aorta and when it does, it is known as an aortic aneurism. Think of this like the bulges that can form in old tires when the rubber weakens or becomes less elastic.

Dimitroulis et al in the *Journal of Vascular Surgery* (2011) showed that in aortic aneurisms, the telomerase activity was less in the endothelium. Interesting, no? We prefer this kind of study in the actual aortic cells of interest because it doesn't rely upon LTL measurement and the false assumption that white blood cells reflect damage of every organ all the time.

I don't know if this is a radical idea but I truly believe that high blood pressure isn't a disease, it's actually the cure! What do I mean by that?

As the arteries become harder and they lose their propulsive force from stem cell aging, the only way to perfuse brain, kidneys and other organs with blood is to excessively tighten the pipes or grow the heart pump stronger. It is like trying to spray your car in the driveway with a hose. If the stream doesn't reach, you kink the hose so the water can reach farther.

The increased blood pressure is therefore the body's compensation to get the stream to where it needs to go. If the arteries were contracting well and propelling blood forward as they were designed to, and if they were rubbery enough to store energy by virtue of the *Windkessel Effect*, then you wouldn't need to clamp down and squeeze a faster stream through a tighter diameter.

In some, but certainly not all patients, we have seen arteries recover their elasticity soon after starting TA-65, in the absence of any other changes in medication or lifestyle.

We will have to wait for a well-designed randomized controlled trial of telomerase activation and hypertension. If this turns out to be related, softer arteries might be resulting in one of the few untoward things that can happen after taking a telomerase activator: dizziness upon standing in patients still persisting on their full strength blood pressure medications.

Blood pressure medications should be tapered if the blood pressure becomes newly normal. This orthostatic hypotension (low blood pressure from standing) is something a qualified telomerase activation medicine specialist would watch for.

So where is the proof that telomere erosion hurts blood vessels? Nzietchueng et al's study looked at vessel health and the telomeres in the cells comprising those vessels (*The Journal of Nutrition, Health & Aging* (2011). They found that diseased veins and arteries had shorter telomeres than the healthy ones. Lacking our stem cell theory of aging, the last sentence of the abstract was obtuse and unwarranted, illustrating my warning not to judge the meal on the after-dinner group photo: "These results also suggest tissue regulation of telomere size by local factors likely related to oxidative stress responses."

For more information on high blood pressure, see Podcast 30 on my YouTube channel, "*drpark65.*"

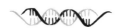

Osteoporosis

Danish scientists, Kveiborg et al did one of the early studies looking at telomere length and bone-generating stem cells called osteoblasts (*Mechanisms of Aging and Development* (1999). As we might predict, younger women had longer osteoblast telomere length than older women (9320 versus 7800 base pairs). The same women had leukocyte telomere length measuring 6760 in the younger and 6420 in the older women. It is worth noting that between the osteoblast stem cell (9320bp) and the white blood cell (6760bp) cell types there was a 2560 base pair difference in length! For the older women there was 1380 base pair difference between the two cell types.

This illustrates my point that LTL does not necessarily bear correlation with telomere length in other cells; in this case, osteoblasts, for example.

Regrettably, the authors made the unfortunate conclusion that telomere length is unrelated to aging because they had received and accepted the axiom that LTL is synonymous with aging. Thankfully, if we ignore the last sentence of the abstract, we can appreciate that the study proved telomere erosion is taking place in osteoporosis. Because they assumed the hoof beats outside were zebras, they were disappointed to not find zebra hair in the street when they went outside.

Interestingly, this bias of study design was duplicated 10 years later by Sanders et al in *The Journal of Bone and Mineral Research* (2009). The authors showed that LTL is not tightly correlated with osteoporosis. They didn't even bother looking for horse hair this time. In other words, they ignored the cells of interest, the osteoblasts. In effect, they proved that tire tread can't predict chassis damage, and that zebra hair can't be found when only horses are present.

In my opinion, there is absolutely no theoretical or practical reason to believe that all other stem cell types would not vary wildly from the leukocyte measurement, in accordance with the stress and replicative senescence of those particular stem cells. For instance, an alcoholic is aging his esophagus and liver more rapidly than other stem cells and so the rate of erosion and accumulation of errors will be faster in stem cells of the esophagus and liver. Likewise, a smoker or coal miner is undergoing constant inflammation and repeated copying of their lung stem cells leading that particular host's "air filter" to age faster than their tire tread.

For more information on osteoporosis, see Podcast 6 on my YouTube channel, "*drpark65.*"

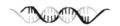

Arthritis

One of the hallmarks of aging, whether in "normal" people or in the accelerated aging of children, is osteoarthritis, or the degeneration of the cushioning cartilage at the surfaces where bone meets bone.

Harbo et al in *Arthritis Research and Therapy* (2012) studied arthritis using a methodology that ignores white blood cells (the tire tread). They looked at cartilage from real human knees and characterized the damage as you got farther from the central lesion. As we would predict from our knowledge of stem cell biology and niches, the closer you were to the central lesion (or the sickest of the hives) the worse was the arthritis, the more senescent were the cells, the shorter were the telomeres, and the higher was the percentage of critically-short telomeres. Critically-short telomeres are sometimes defined as those with less than 1500 base pairs, a possible threshold equivalent to being functionally naked or uncapped.

But was this statistically significant? Absolutely! In fact, the statistical probability of randomly finding these differences in the 21 patients studied was 1 in a million for arthritis grade, 2 in a million for senescence, 4 in a million for telomere length, and 7 in a thousand for critically-short telomeres.

For more information on arthritis, see Podcast 30 on my YouTube channel, "*drpark65*."

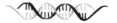

AIDS is Immune Aging and Aging Brings a Form of AIDS

Your body is like the Roman Empire. There are enemies at the frontiers and enemies from within. In order to stay intact, your legions need to protect you from invaders such as bacteria, viruses, and weird particles on your skin and in the respiratory and gastrointestinal systems. It also needs to respond to threats from within, such as cancer, yeast, and wart and herpes-like viruses hiding inside your cells.

Your immune system creatively and actively responds to these new threats using the "B" and the "T" white blood cells systems.

"B" stands for bone marrow and these cells are responsible for generating the antibodies, which are tiny specific, y-shaped molecules that bind and mark for destruction things like a polio virus or a tetanus toxin. But B-cells require T-cells to coordinate and to mobilize quickly.

"T" stands for the thymus, which is a small fatty organ laying atop your breastplate. It is there that your T-cells learn to recognize the host but are destroyed if they are overly aggressive to the self. If T-cells make it through this cellular "West Point Academy" they are ready to respond to new threats and circulate, just waiting to suppress any would-be infections or cancers.

Brief digression: if you've ever seen Stanley Kubrick's movie, *Full Metal Jacket* (Warner Brothers, 1987) then you know what you need to know about autoimmune diseases. Like T-Cells in the thymus, the recruits in that movie were specifically selected and trained to kill, working together as a unit of soldiers. But one of the overweight recruits that they called "Gomer Pyle" became overly aggressive after severe bullying and became a psychotic killer. In basic training, overly aggressive cadets need to be weeded out.

Similarly, the failure to weed out overly aggressive T-cells before leaving the thymus results in autoimmune disease.

Even Galen, the father of Western Medicine who lived from 129-200 CE, recognized that the thymus withers with age. This is in direct correlation to our deterioration of immune health and can be measured by checking a cell surface "freshness" marker called CD28 (cellular differentiation 28). A CD28 positive cell is one that can still respond to new threats, like a blank key that has yet to be cut to fit a new lock.

As we age, there is an increase in the percentage of CD28 absent also known as CD28(-) (read as "CD28 negative") T-cells. This indicates cells that are burned-out and that will not be able to respond to new threats. In both Acquired Immune Deficiency Syndrome (AIDS) caused by a virus and immune deficiency associated with aging, we develop immune deficiency that can be measured by the increase of CD28 negative cells which I believe is brought about by telomere shortening from replicative senescence.

Harley et al in *Rejuvenation Research* (2009), looked at the cohort of pioneers to first take TA-65 and found that after starting a TA program, the percentage of burned-out CD28 negative cells fell dramatically, especially if the person was CMV (cytomegalovirus) infected. In addition, the percentage of cells with short telomeres (defined here as <4000 base pairs) decreased after TA-65 ingestion. I believe that TA-induced apoptosis may have facilitated both these changes. Apoptosis, or "programmed cell death", will be discussed in Chapter 9: "Telomerase activation medicine."

The second way TA may help immune function is also described in that upcoming chapter as competitive advantage or stochastic improvement. It is that precise idea that was proven by

Fauce et al in *The Journal of Immunology* (2008). They took a telomerase activator discovered by the Geron Corporation and found that because of telomerase activation, the T-cells, especially HIV-infected ones, were able to function, reproduce, and protect themselves better. Specific blockage of telomerase activation negated this effect proving it was the telomerase activation itself that was likely responsible.

That study was co-authored by the leading expert in this field, Dr. Rita Effros of the UCLA Geffen School of Medicine. She is the leading expert in the senescence of the immune system and my patients undergoing telomerase activation medicine testing have access to these CD28 measurements.

As we learn more, we realize that immune senescence and aging may be a chicken and egg causation quandary. Chronic, incurable infections such as CMV, the cytomegalovirus, may be grinding down our systems like Barbarians at the gate. That is why someone as physically intact as Jack LaLanne could be overwhelmed by the common cold. He had simply exhausted all his blank keys, or CD28 positive T-cells

For more information on the immune system, please see my Podcast 36 on my YouTube channel *"drpark65."*

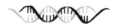

Cancer is Usually from Shortening of Telomeres

Willeit et al published a very important and elegant study looking at 787 patients prospectively for a 10-year period, in *The Journal of the American Medical Association* (2010). With 100% follow-up of their clinical histories and blood samples, 12% of the patients developed cancer. For both genders and all cancer types, the rate of cancer and the aggressiveness of their disease were directly proportional to the degree of telomere shortening the cells had undergone. One disease, Lady Godiva, checkmate.

To quote the pithy Professor Gump: "and that's all I have to say about that."

We could engage in a debate citing a vast and apparently conflicting literature looking at telomere length and cancers of every type. But let us remember Professor David Deutsche wants us to choose "hard-to-vary" explanations.

I have already explained that telomerase activity in cancer cells is a retained trait of stemness but in fairness, there is also an alternative lengthening of telomeres (ALT for short) that can occur in cancer cells. This type of lengthening involves crossover from neighboring telomeres and it also allows for lengthening, even in the absence of telomerase activity.

When it comes to looking at the telomeres of existing cancers, I think long versus short telomeres is a false dichotomy and an oversimplification. I believe that the reason some studies show that tumors possess lengthened telomeres is that they are like freaky zombies.

The telomerase engine and/or the ALT mechanism continues to operate normally even after the initial carcinogenic changes occurred. The bartender just keeps filling up those shot glasses, or lengthening all telomeres, even after critical shortening, inappropriate splicing, and chromosomal mutations have created the cancer.

When you look at the actual chromosomes from cancers under a microscope, they are indeed bizarre, recombined, and chopped up in an infinite variety of ways.

But there are also often abnormally long telomeres in those chromosomes making interpretation based upon median telomere length data confusing. Sadly, our easy-to-vary but vast scientific literature regarding telomeres has mostly just proven that if you ask the wrong question, you'll get an unhelpful answer.

Incidentally, the same holds true for older people with abnormally long LTL before taking a TA. Increased median length alone may not indicate health so much as overgrowth and poorly trimmed telomeres. That is why the use of percentage of critically-shortened telomeres provided by the Life Length test is so helpful. In my older patients, if the median telomere length drops initially but the percentage of critically-shortened telomeres also drops, I am happy. Even though my patients are usually displeased by the shortened length, that change may represent a destruction of aberrant stem cells by apoptosis and the increased health of the cell populations as a whole.

Think of it as being like body weight. If I told you a person was 150 pounds, could you tell me how healthy they were? Probably not. You would need to know the gender, height, body composition, number of limbs, nutritional and fluid balance, the recent fluctuations and all their other health and disease conditions.

We need to appreciate that mutation takes place at the individual telomere level. And consider that every one of the 184 telomeres in each of your billions of stem cells in your body is shortening and lengthening at its own pace. To the untrained inspector of prisoners of war, it may seem that the average hair length of the telomeres indicates that the cells are well-treated and healthy. If so, they are basing it upon their recollection of the musical, *Hair*, in which hair length was a proxy for something vibrant and creative. But they need to check the teeth, look for lice, and watch for Morse code in the eye-blinking before drawing any conclusions.

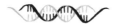

A New Paradigm for Cancer Prevention and Treatment

Almost everything you know about cancer is wrong. That's not your fault.

You might think cancer is hereditary, rare, robust and deadly. Like truth, beauty, and aging, the term "cancer" is also hopelessly vague and unhelpful. That is because all pre-cancers, low malignant potential cancers, in-situ (non-traveling) cancers, and all the "regular" cancers overlap in their normal versus abnormal behaviors.

The activity of telomerase, as we have already discussed, may be an artifact of stemness, reflecting the cancer queen bee stem cell's origins from Krypton (see Chapter 5: "Stem Cells" if you don't quite grasp that reference).

Other behaviors that vary include contact inhibition, which is the ability to be suppressed by their neighbors and not overgrow their allotted elbowroom. The lack of contact inhibition allows for invading and disseminating beyond that boundary- a process called metastasis.

The truth is that cancer is usually not hereditary unless you carry only a single working copy of a gene encoding an enzyme like p53, that is supposed to monitor for cell mutation. Cancer is the inevitable consequence of repeated copying in the presence of inadequate telomerase activity and it can occur from random mutations as well.

Cancer is common and may have already occurred billions of times in your body. It was handled by your immune system, 'burned out' from replicative senescence or most likely, became so damaged from repeated copying and mutation that it was no longer viable.

Cancer is not always robust and is often fragile. These are damaged cells to begin with and although we cannot currently identify them, there may be instances where the body would have naturally rid itself of cancer if we didn't poison the immune system and burn the tissues.

Cancer is not always deadly. At autopsy for death from other causes, Yin et al in the *Journal of Urology* (2008) found that 46% percent of men 70 years and above had undiagnosed prostate cancer. Skin cancer can also remain premalignant and even malignant for quite some time before losing contact inhibition and behaving badly.

To understand my new paradigm for cancer prevention or treatment, I made a diagram showing our current methods, illustrated as a pyramid above the surface, balancing on its point. But there is one under the surface, which I would call the unrecognized "pyramid of cancer prevention."

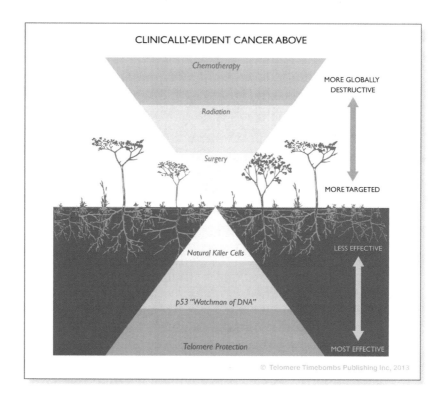

CLINICALLY-EVIDENT CANCER ABOVE

Chemotherapy

MORE GLOBALLY DESTRUCTIVE

Radiation

Surgery

MORE TARGETED

Natural Killer Cells

LESS EFFECTIVE

p53 "Watchman of DNA"

Telomere Protection

MOST EFFECTIVE

© Telomere Timebombs Publishing Inc, 2013

It is better to prevent cancer than to treat it

The sole medical paradigm now is the one above ground in the illustration. In that model, Cancer is treated by several methods. The first tier is targeted surgical removal, which is often, but not always, the least destructive and most effective.

The second wider tier of radiation therapy carries with it more collateral damage to healthy native tissues, other adjacent organs, and circulating blood cells as well.

The most damaging and globally destructive treatment used is chemotherapy, whose aim is to poison to all cells, especially the rapidly-reproducing ones. That is akin to Agent Orange; it is like a high altitude neutron bomb that indiscriminately kills everything from 10,000 feet.

Thankfully, scientists have developed monoclonal antibodies with poison attached that may act more like magic bullets. But the "old school" chemo is like trying to solve a hostage crisis by pumping poison gas or narcotics into the air ventilation system.

If you really understand what chemo does, then you shouldn't be surprised that one of the worst side effects is new cancers from all the mutations you introduce into stem cells. Another of the many unfortunate side effects of poisoning with chemo is the brain fog caused by inducing mutations in the neural stem cells.

Chemotherapy works because it intentionally yet randomly writes more DNA errors and impairs cell division. It still depends upon each cell's apoptosis program to kick in as the drugs to not "know" how to kill. Hayashi et al in *Nature Structure & Molecular Biology* (2012) showed that chemotherapy was increasing damage to telomeres and in the presence of p53, this allowed for cell apoptosis. Why further damage already damaged cells to make them kill themselves when we could have just prevented the problem to begin with?

That brings us to the upward facing pyramid of cancer prevention below the surface. I think this is the first time anyone has conceptualized it in this way, but I can't claim any original thinking here because everything about this idea is common knowledge. I'm just the little kid pointing out the obvious nakedness of the Emperor and making a picture to illustrate the hard-to-vary truths of cancer.

Why would the wide base and the most important aspect of cancer prevention be the maintenance of telomeres? Well, it should be self-evident to you by now that if the ends never shorten, the inappropriately spliced double chromosomes never form, the chromosomes don't get torn up and progressively worse, and therefore the cancer doesn't develop.

The second layer of the prevention pyramid is our watchman of the genome in every cell, the p53 enzyme, which is really a proxy for the many checking mechanisms. Suffice it to say this is the "always-on" system of self-checking and self-destruction that is a primary mission of each and every cell, not just the stem cells.

At the top of the pyramid are the special T-cells known as the Natural Killer Cells. These cells are constantly circulating and are able to recognize and destroy cancer cells naturally, without the need to "learn" the threat as with viruses and without the help of radiation and chemotherapy.

So to summarize this lengthy chapter, a vast scientific literature validates the premise of what I call "telomerase activation medicine." There is truly only one disease with many faces, or one rider with many steeds: the accumulation of genetic damage from telomere erosion in stem cells. Recall that genetic damage in non-stem cells is irrelevant because it will burn out and is non-immortal because there is no telomerase activity.

Disease is not an accident or a genetic curse as most believe, but rather like rust or friction in car parts. You wouldn't take your car into the dealer at 300,000 miles and remark that "nobody in my family ever had to replace a muffler." Yet that is exactly what most people think when they get colon cancer despite not having a family history for that condition.

Actually, if you could survive every disease and replace organs with new ones, by age 300 you would have contracted nearly every disease. By replacement with your own custom-differentiated, personalized stem cell-derived organs, you would have already gone blind and gotten new eyes, lost your hearing and had your inner ears' cochleas replaced, had kidney failure and swapped out those 'beans' many times, and developed and rid yourself of cancer of everything.

Now if telomere erosion can be halted with telomerase activity, as with Henrietta Lacks' immortal cervical cancer cells, then maybe you can run your original parts much longer. Future telomerase activation medicine will reveal which parts have longer lives and which need more frequent changing (like a steering wheel versus an oil filter).

But don't forget the good news of how the body is able to rid itself of damaged stem cells with apoptosis and replace them with newer refurbished parts from mesenchymal stem cells (see Chapter 5: "Stem Cells").

If I have done my job, you should be flabbergasted. I am. Why is it that nobody is screaming the simple and universal truth that telomere erosion is at the center of all diseases, when it is clearly a central focus of all those scientists in all those separate "wheel inventing" laboratories around the world?

Buckminster Fuller said: "You never change things by fighting the existing reality. To change something, build a new model that makes the existing model obsolete." Hopefully, my simple stem cell theory of disease and aging will do just that.

In the next chapter, we will discuss the very thing that I don't truly believe in: aging.

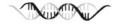

7

AGING SLOW, FAST, AND NOT AT ALL

"Beauty is truth, truth beauty," – that is all
Ye know on earth, and all ye need to know."
— John Keats

"I shall not today attempt further to define the
kinds of material I understand to be embraced
within that shorthand description ["hard-core
pornography"]; and perhaps I could never
*succeed in intelligibly doing so. But **I know it***
***when I see it**, and the motion picture involved in*
this case is not that."
—Justice Potter Stewart

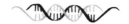

Remember when I said I don't believe in aging? It's true. But don't we all just "know it when we see it?" In this chapter, our goals are to examine the nature of accelerated and decelerated "aging," find out why the Bible agrees with science regarding our maximum lifespan, and make the case for aging in reverse.

I believe the concept of aging is so inextricably linked with our subjective reality, that it is an unassailable truth and tautology (an argument where the conclusion is essentially the premise). I don't like unassailable truths and I like to shoot arrows of "Why?" at them.

When you think about it, aging is a very abstract concept like truth, beauty, or pornography that is way too easy-to-vary to be a good explanation or robust concept. Keats wasn't very helpful defining the first two and Justice Potter Stewart was even less so with his most famous quote (above).

I challenge you to act as the supreme judge of whether you believe in aging. For example, and not just as an academic exercise, consider that if you thaw an embryo from 10 years ago that has been metabolically inactive, that the baby born now could be considered almost 11 years old? Or if a person exercises, changes their lifestyle, and achieves a more youthful physiology, are they not aging backwards? Inversely, if a person is caring for a dying spouse or is elected President of the United States, do they not age more rapidly?

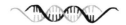

Aging Slowly: It's Not Magic, it's Maintenance

Irving Gordon of Long Island, NY has cared for his Volvo P1800 to the point of 3 million miles. It isn't magic, it's maintenance. So is that beloved car forty-something years old, 3 million miles old, or brand new because it has brand-new replacement parts? It is said that none of your cells are the same from 7 years ago. I don't know if I believe that but I literally bet my life that if you could keep telomeres from eroding, you would age a lot slower.

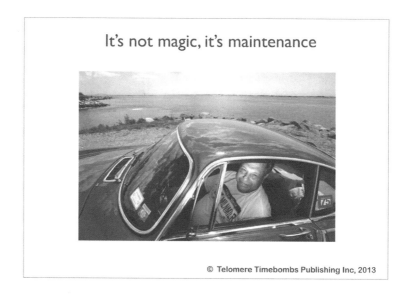

It's not magic, it's maintenance

© Telomere Timebombs Publishing Inc, 2013

Your body can be maintained like a car

So if we don't measure age by trips around the sun, what is the alternative? The answer comes from Dr. Joseph Rafaelle, the original consultant to Telomerase Activation Sciences, Inc. T.A. Sciences® is the maker of the world's first safe telomerase activator that we will discuss in the next chapter. Dr. Rafaelle has created something called a PhysioAge™ measurement.

Your PhysioAge is based on their proprietary, best-fit modeling that can include measurements of skin elasticity, lung capacity, arterial compliance, mental acuity, immune function, and leukocyte telomere measurements. This is the gold standard that I use in my practice and these measurements provide invaluable information as to how our patients are doing as they grow younger.

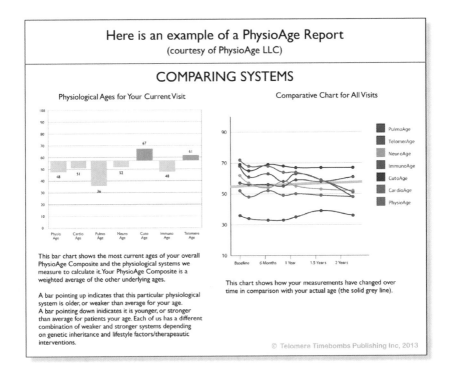

Here is an example of a PhysioAge Report
(courtesy of PhysioAge LLC)

You can measure your biological age using a PhysioAge exam

Now I already said that I consider LTL to be like checking tire tread and that it can't be used as a proxy for all organs. What we truly need is a Star Trek-type "tricorder" to measure the telomere damage in all cells, by niche, and color-code them. Even better would be to show the exact damage to the individual chromosomes. Actually, a color coding study of telomere lengths was done by Blasco's lab as: "The longest telomeres: a general signature of adult stem cell compartments." Flores et al. *Genes & Development,* (2008). They showed that the longest telomeres were found nearest to the fountains of stem cell regeneration in all organs that need to copy a lot, like hair, small intestines, testes, the cornea, and the brain.

So when a stem cell dies in a nearby niche, like a pigment-generating melanocyte coloring a hair follicle, perhaps a locally-generated stem cell rather than an itinerant mesenchymal stem cell queen bee is the likely source of replacement stem cells.

If telomerase activation is like routine scheduled car maintenance, then how can we increase telomerase activity and live longer? You already know the answer but there is a study proving what we all know from common sense. Nobel Prize winner, Professor Elizabeth Blackburn, and Dr. Dean Ornish collaborated on a study showing changes in behaviors such as diet, exercise, sleep, and stress reduction through meditation are all associated with increased telomerase activity, lower cholesterol, and lower stress. See Ornish et al in *Lancet Oncology* (2008). Perhaps all the good things people do to stay young are somehow mediated through telomerase activity?

What is the evidence that an increase in telomerase is associated with increased lifespan? One study from the Albert Einstein School of Medicine studied Ashkenazi centenarians, or people living to be 100 (Atzmon et al, *Proceedings of the National Academy of Sciences* (2009). They found that centenarians had an unusually high telomerase activity suggesting again that my telomere/stem cell theory of aging is "hard-to-vary."

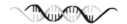

Telomere Measurements: It's Not Just About Length

If we forget the tricorder and pretend that LTL is a direct measurement of a person's true genetic age, then I should be extremely pleased! After taking a TA for over five years, my genetic age is like that of a teenager. As you will see, the measurement dropped initially, then rose while increasing the dose of TA-65, dropped when I couldn't afford to take it, and then increased beyond baseline when I resumed.

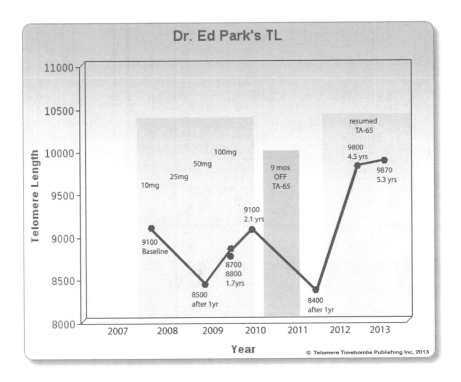

My telomere length is getting longer, not shorter

There are several labs offering blood testing and two involving saliva that can quantify your own median, not average, telomere length in your white blood cells. We use median, because unusually long or short telomeres could disproportionately affect our estimates. Just like median house price is a better measurement if you live in the neighborhood of someone like Bill Gates.

There are a few labs that measure median leukocyte telomere length in the United States but I prefer tests that quantify the critically-shortened telomeres. Life Length is a company that offers such a blood test throughout the US, Canada, and most of Europe. There is another company called TeloME that also measures critically-shortened telomeres from a saliva sample.

The discoverer of TA-65 and one of the leading researchers into telomerase activation and telomere biology, Dr. Cal Harley, also founded a company called Telome Health that offers an affordable and highly validated test of median telomere length from saliva testing.

For more information regarding telomere measurements, please see my Podcast 37 on my YouTube channel "*drpark65*."

So really, "aging" can be considered mental shorthand that we use to describe multiple concepts. First, it represents the accumulation of damage in the cells and organs that generally and progressively afflicts us as we travel forward in time.

Second, aging signifies the functional loss of our capabilities that we dread and mourn. And finally, it is a sort of death sentence that we accept, like a yoke on an ox, although the fact that you are reading this book means the yoke may no longer be on you.

Now you might feel sad for a kid dying of old age at 12 years because you think everyone has the right to die at 80, right? Wrong. You might believe that the universe or God will punish you for wanting and achieving a lifespan of hundreds of healthy years, right? Why? Is the Volvo Corporation going to strike Irving Gordon down with wrathful vengeance for maintaining his automobile with routine maintenance and parts? On the contrary, they love the guy!

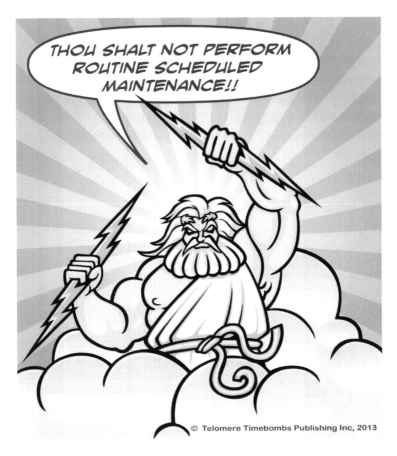

Would you consider it a sin to change your oil?

I believe that Irv holds a double standard when it comes to his car versus his body. If you had asked him in 1966 how many thousands of miles he would put on his new car, he would have told you maybe a hundred. How wrong he would have been. But today, if you ask Mr. Gordon, now aged 73, how long he can live in his current body, he might sheepishly say one hundred again. But Irv, buddy! Your body is just like your car!

Please grasp this basic principle now: telomere erosion from replicative senescence is always on, but so is telomerase reverse transcription and lengthening.

The length of your telomeres is dynamic. We step on the analogy clutch and run through your choice of gears. Aging, as determined by shortening/lengthening of telomeres, is like: 1) Pouring water into a bucket with a hole in it; 2) Walking up an escalator that is taking you down; 3) Paddling up a river against the current; 4) Growing your hair or your lawn while also needing to cut them; 5) Splicing more fuse length onto the stick of dynamite that is lit and burning on both ends; or 6) A bartender constantly refilling rows of shot glasses being sipped at by endless patrons.

My personal leukocyte telomere lengths over the last six years show that LTL is always in flux and suggest that a telomerase activator can accelerate the pouring of water, speed of running back up the escalator, growth rate of your grass or hair, or your efficiency of adding fuse length to the dynamite.

Take home lesson? As Neil Young warned us, "rust never sleeps." But then again, neither do the telomerase micromachines. That is why the lengths on all the stem cells' telomeres are dynamically changing. In contrast, because they lack telomerase activity, non-stem cells' telomeres can only erode.

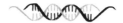

Accelerated Aging is Accelerated Genetic Damage in Stem Cells

If you want proof that telomere erosion is the most important factor in aging, we only need to look at progeria ("towards aging") or the premature aging syndromes in those "Make-A-Wish

Foundation" kids that die at age 12 with wrinkles, arthritis, osteoporosis and heart disease. They have gone around the sun only 12 times, but unlike their peers, their telomeres, stem cells, organs, and diseases are largely indistinguishable from those of 80-year-olds.

There are different types of accelerated aging but for the most part, they usually involve failure of DNA maintenance and repair. The classic natural model of accelerated aging is known as dyskeratosis congenita. "Congenita" means it is inherited, and "dyskeratosis" means the poor growth and maintenance keratin-containing structures, such as the skin, hair, and nails.

The reason for the dyskeratosis is that skin, hair, and nails function in a constantly regenerating way. So the Lady Godiva of replicative senescence "rides" those types preferentially, resulting in genetic damage that leads to impaired stem cell integrity, proliferation, and migration out to their niches.

Thankfully, scientists have worked out the mechanics of this disease and they have found that often, certain mutations in one of the copies of the dyskerin gene or its paired TERC gene (telomerase RNA component) are to blame (see Chapter 4: "Telomerase"). This half-gene dosage is known as haploid or heterozygous for the wild type because the other copy is a non-functional mutant. Because you have less telomerase activity, you simply can't maintain your telomeres. Loss of heterozygosity in that instance would render the cell line unsustainable.

But to say that an abnormal copy of the dyskerin gene on one of your two chromosomes causes poor telomerase activity is like saying having one glass eye causes poor vision.

Gene dosage is an important concept to understand. A cell's "gene dosage" refers to the number of copies of a gene it has. One copy per chromosome and one chromosome from each parent means two copies is what is known as a full, diploid gene dosage. Why is that important? Quite simply, the higher the gene dosage of telomerase, the more telomerase activity you get. And based on the Ashkenazi study, the natural experiment of dyskeratosis congenita, and common sense, telomerase activity is strongly correlated with increased longevity.

That is usually what is meant when we say a person is a "carrier" for a disease. You have one functioning copy but there is no decent backup copy. The system usually has two copies of a gene or a DIPLOID dosage; it's kind of like having two kidneys so that if one is gone, you still can function.

If a mutation occurs in the only remaining normal, wild-type copy, we achieve what is called "loss of heterozygosity." That is a cumbersome way of saying your only good kidney just died and now you have two bad copies, or non wild-type versions of the gene in question.

Brief digression: did you know that oncogenes don't cause cancer but instead prevent it? The genes that predispose to high rates of cancer are always involved in DNA repair, maintenance, and apoptosis. Contrary to what most people believe, the problem isn't having the oncogene, it is having only one good copy of the normal gene, or a haploid gene dosage.

How counterintuitive is that? To call a BRCA1 or BRCA2 gene a "cancer gene" is like calling a police force at half-strength a crime promoter. There are many ways an oncogene can be defective and sadly, people routinely have their breasts and ovaries removed because of their cells carrying an abnormal variant. But there is always one remaining normal oncogene still working in those cells tossed into the surgical specimen bucket. Having one abnormal oncogene is like having one cup of motor oil and one cup of orange juice for breakfast. You aren't going to drink the oil and would prefer having two glasses of orange juice. But hey, you still have the one glass of orange juice to drink.

Just as the manner in which a bad kidney died isn't relevant, so the sequence of mutations only matter if you "own" them and profit from testing for them. A good clinician knows not to order tests unless the proposed tests would change management and since I don't believe in preventative or prophylactic surgery, I don't often recommend this type of testing. Being a BRCA carrier simply means you are heterozygous for that bad gene and if your one good copy is lost, there might be trouble. Incidentally, the BRCA1 and BRCA2 genes are both implicated in telomere maintenance. There we have more hard-to-vary evidence that telomere dysfunction is at the heart of why we develop cancer.

Back to progeria now. It turns out that dyskeratosis congenita can also be caused by a decreased gene dosage in other genes involving the telomerase enzyme (TERT,) telomerase RNA component (TERC) and TINF2 (a protein needed for functioning of the micromachine "lock and key").

Thus, nature has already done multiple versions of the experiment proving beyond a doubt that any decrease in telomerase activity, by any mechanism, will yield you the same disease: accelerated and premature aging.

If you possess two copies all the required genes in this modern world, you are probably going to make it to 80 years. That is the current, programmed average lifespan. But what would happen if you had three or four copies of all the components needed for telomerase activity? Or what if you could maximize, using a telomerase activator, the functioning of the two copies that you already have? Would that allow you to live hundreds of years, just as Methuselah is reputed to have lived 969 years?

Now is a good time to address the elephant in the room. If you have made it to this part of the book, you should be starting to accept that what we know as aging is simply the accumulation of preventable and apoptotically-correctable damage in stem cells. Perhaps you have occasionally let your mind wander off and ask "Gee, I wonder how more years of healthy life I could have if this is all true?"

When we consider what anti-aging guru and scientist Aubrey de Grey has called "negligible senescence," we start to engage in conjecture to which only science fiction can do justice. I mentioned in Chapter 2: "My hero's journey," about how I became a screenwriter and wrote *Maximum Lifespan*. That story addresses negligible senescence in several ways.

In *Maximum Lifespan*, a scientist secretly clones himself into his two "sons" and plans to download his consciousness into the healthy one's body to escape dying. If you successfully could do that, is it still "you" that exists in another person's body? Problems of a metaphysical nature arise.

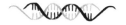

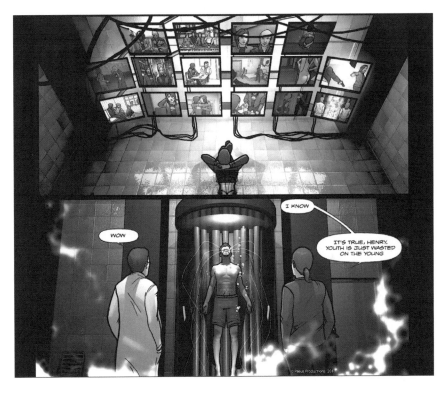

Evil dad reviews his son's memories after hijacking his body

According to the Bible, it might appear that God didn't care for humans living so long. So perhaps the Almighty resolved to decrease the telomerase activity of humans, made it rain for 40 days and 40 nights, and reengineered the species away from 900+ trips around the sun.

> *Days of our years, in them are seventy years, and if, by reason of might, eighty years, Yet is their enlargement labour and vanity, For it hath been cut off hastily, and we fly away.*
> — Psalm 90:10, New King James Version

Why does the survival curve (the percentage of people still alive at a given age) look like a side view of Niagara Falls? That is because of something I call the "Orville Redenbacher® effect." When you are cooking microwave popcorn, it looks like nothing is going on for a minute and then the kernels start popping. All stem cells throughout your body are constantly accumulating their own damage so at some point, often triggered by an unusually stressful time when telomerase activity can't keep up, a person will manifests more than one disease in a short period of time, such as diabetes, high blood pressure, and cancer. As Gilda Radner's *Saturday Night Live* character, "Roseanne Roseanannadanna" would always complain, "If it's not one thing, it's another!"

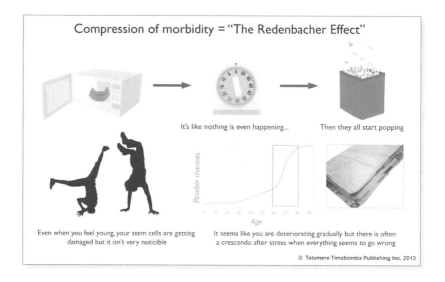

"If it's not one thing, it's another"

The goal of telomerase activation medicine is to shift the curve to the right, so your Redenbacher effect takes place at 90 or 110 or perhaps even later. And this is what my patients want also. They always tell me, "When it's my time to go, that's fine; but I want to be as healthy as possible until then." That is like making the curve into a cliff. Although the curve represents a population, it might just as well represent the serious disease(s) that you accumulate suddenly, just prior to death.

As for the maximum human lifespan, leading researcher Dr. L. Stephen Coles of UCLA's Gerontology Research Group agrees with the Bible that 120 is the limit:

> *And the Lord said, My spirit shall not always strive with man, for that he also is flesh: yet his days shall be a <u>hundred and twenty years</u>.*
>
> — Genesis 6:3, New King James Version

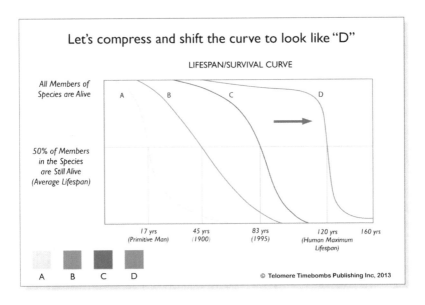

Maximum lifespan is set in stone,
but not if telomerase is increased

That is 100% correct. In 2013, we have complete agreement between science and the Bible. When he started keeping track of people living past 110 (supercentenarians) thirty years ago, Dr. Coles assumed that by now, more people would be breaking the 120 barrier. Alas, environmental and medical progress has utterly failed to shift the curve; it would appear that 120 is the maximum when it comes to our limits of longevity.

At least that used to be the case until TA-65 was discovered.

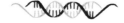

8

TELOMERASE ACTIVATORS

The Grail Knight, speaking to Indiana Jones right before choosing his cup:

"You must choose, but choose wisely. For as the true Grail will bring you life, the false Grail will take it from you."
—*Indiana Jones and the Last Crusade*
(Paramount Pictures, 1989)

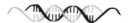

A telomerase activator can theoretically cure aging and in fact, I am confident that is exactly what it does. That is a very big deal. In a strange case of art prefiguring life, that discovery was one of many things from my graphic novel, *Maximum Lifespan,* which came to fruition in the real world. I had already imagined a world with telomerase activators and that is why I jumped at the chance to become the 19th person in the world to regularly ingest a real one.

I reviewed the safety data before beginning but it was still a pretty big leap of faith. Would it be safe? Were fears about cancer going to be justified? I had already lost my father and my boys needed a father, so I needed to be cautious.

This chapter will discuss the origins and significance of the world's first safe and effective telomerase activator, TA-65. But before I tell you the story of how TA-65 came into existence, let us wax philosophically about the concept of time for just a moment.

The tapestry of every human life is spun from feelings, thoughts, and events and is constantly being woven into a more or less coherent story. Embedded deep within our personal, collective, and universal souls is the concept of time and its meaning. Without time, stitches would be woven without order and we have only yarn without patterns or meaning.

It may sound strange, but as in the case of aging, I literally don't believe in time. Time is merely a tool that mankind invented in order to parse out and organize reality. It is not, as some suggest, a "fourth dimension." Religion at its most profound level again agrees with theoretical physics in this regard. It is entirely possible that despite our protestations, nothing is ever "happening" and that the universe or many universes just exist, without creation, living and destruction (symbolized by the Hindu trinity of Brahma, Vishnu, and Shiva).

That is not to say that universe is impersonal, or that consciousness is not the force driving it. Stating the obvious: the egg can't create the egg. Even if there is a universal God for a physical universe, there will always be, by definition, something bigger and smaller in scale.

When we reflect upon our own lives, it is always, inextricably, understood in the context of the river of time. This river's undercurrents and eddies we call birthdays, funerals, graduations, marriages, pay periods, and alarm clocks. You likely have picked up this book in order to try to paddle back upstream the river of longevity but probably didn't consider the possibility of parking your canoe on a sand bar and just enjoying the view as others huff and puff their way against the raging waters.

Again, I sincerely believe that aging has now been made obsolete by the discovery and use of a single molecule telomerase activator that people are taking. This chapter's dilemma: "If all this is true, should I consider trying TA-65 myself?" In order to answer that, I will describe how TA-65 came into existence so that, as the Grail Knight cautioned Indiana Jones, you can "choose wisely."

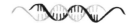

Remove the "Non" for Just this Chapter of Non-fiction
The majority of people to whom I explain TA become closed off mentally and unable to process rationally above the din of their own internal turmoil. In my experience, this notion is so painful and unpleasant because it appears to be mocking and cruel. If that is the case with you, I recommend that you treat this entire chapter as fiction. Pretend that it's all a big joke or a fantasy. After reading it, you can look it up on the internet, but please don't take on the responsibility of having to judge the veracity of a single word I'm saying because that would slow you down.

I wrote this book, *Telomere Timebombs,* in order to explain telomere biology but also to introduce you to the world's first scientifically-proven, commercially-available telomerase activator, TA-65. As a direct result of taking TA-65, my life, my health, and my career have been transformed. That is because of the amazing and undeniable benefits my patients and I have enjoyed since 2007, the year it was brought to market.

What is TA-65? The identity of TA-65 is a proprietary matter and one that you can research. T.A. Sciences Inc. is the manufacturer and they state that it is a single molecule derived from a Chinese medicinal herb known as Astragalus. Just as the anti-cancer drug, Taxol, is a single molecule (which happens to be derived from the bark of the Pacific Yew Tree) you need to extract the rare molecule of TA-65 from the Astragalus root and discard everything else.

Taking intravenous Pacific Yew Tree bark for cancer or capsules of ground of Astragalus for telomerase activation would be like buying an ounce of dirt instead of an ounce of gold from the general store. It's not the same thing. The TA-65 molecule occurs in such small amounts that you need thousands of pounds of root material to make one person's supply for a year.

Because the molecule cannot be synthesized and must be extracted, and because Astragalus needs to be grown, it is a commodity and the cost of its production is high. The price will come down when more Astragalus is grown, the yield is increased, or scientists will splice the necessary genes into another plant that is mass produced.

Astragalus has been known in traditional Chinese medicine for thousands of years as *Huang qi* (pronounced "hwang chee") and was considered a part of the "heaven class" of *Qi* (life force) tonifying, or strengthening herbs. That means it increases life force and is also thought to improve immunity.

A biotech company called the Geron Corporation located in Menlo Park, has always been at the forefront of studying telomeres and the telomerase enzyme since its founding in 1990. Noel Thomas Patton, the founder of T.A. Sciences, was passionate about longevity and had followed the efforts of the Geron Corporation closely. He was instrumental in introducing scientists from East Asia to scientists at the Geron Corporation. Because it is possible to introduce a single substance into a dish with Henrietta Lacks' immortal HeLA cells and then measure the telomerase activity, the plan was to extract and test individual molecules in search of a magical fountain of youth.

Eventually, that search lead to the discovery of the TA-65 molecule in 2001. By the way, the 'TA' stands for telomerase activator and I'm told by Mr. Patton that '65' refers to the age of forced retirement that is currently most popular. It is imperative to understand that rather than being happenstance or a cure in search of a disease, like resveratrol, the discovery was the direct result of meticulous search, like finding a needle in many stacks of hay.

The US Patent 7,846,904 B2 was granted in 2010 to the Geron Corporation for the use of Astragalus-derived molecules for telomerase activation, six years after its initial filing. Listed among its "inventors" is Calvin Harley, the Chief Scientific Officer of Geron for many years, and five others.

Noel Patton negotiated to obtain the sole rights to distribute the TA-65 molecule for nutraceutical use. Before it could be sold however, meticulous safety testing was performed by T.A. Sciences. I reviewed all these unpublished safety data before taking TA-65 in 2007. I had two small children and was not about to take unnecessary chances.

First, they determined that there was no potential to mutate bacteria using a standard test called the Ames Assay. Secondly, using high-dose single intravenous injection into test animals for toxicity and then examining them at autopsy, it was shown that the molecule was extremely safe even at high doses that would never be taken by humans.

Finally, they took human tumors and grafted onto the backs of immune-compromised mice. The administration of TA-65 did not cause those existing human tumors to grow any faster than when the TA-65 had not been given.

In 2005, T.A. Sciences completed a non-published but randomized controlled trial of TA-65 in human subjects. A randomized controlled trial is a powerful tool used by scientists in which half of the test subjects receive an intervention such as ingesting TA-65, and the other half do not. Because neither the subjects nor the people measuring the results know who is getting the intervention, any statistically abnormal results are deemed to be meaningful. Because they are divided randomly, unknown factors that may have an influenced test results are presumed to be irrelevant because of the randomization.

The results showed improvements in the immune system, vision, male sexual performance, and skin elasticity in the subjects who were given TA-65. As we will discuss in the next chapter, my clinical experience bears out most of this as well.

On July 7, 2007 (note the date of 7/7/7 when humanity hit the jackpot), T.A. Sciences Corporation announced the availability of TA-65 to the public. I stumbled upon this announcement in Fall 2007, did my due diligence about how it came to market, was allowed to see its safety and efficacy data, and then flew out to New York City to start the "Patton Protocol," which is the name for the way to ingest the TA-65 under monitored supervision.

Dr. Joseph Rafaelle, a Park Avenue anti-aging specialist, had worked with T.A. Sciences to develop a series of tests that comprise the "Patton Protocol" under which the TA-65 is administered. Because of my incredible good fortune in stock options trading, the $25,000 a year didn't seem like too much money to see whether immortality was truly possible using this new technology.

I met with Noel and he seemed surprised that a 39-year-old OB/GYN would want to take an anti-aging pill. A year later, I asked to be the first physician outside of T.A. Sciences to be licensed to sell it, after so many of my patients had rhetorically asked me "What are you taking?"

In order to sell TA-65, I had to provide the full Patton Protocol, which meant that I had to purchase $20,000 of testing equipment and pay a $30,000 annual licensing fee for the first year. The vast majority of patients purchased directly from T.A. Sciences and the numbers of competing physicians grew exponentially, so it would be three years before I could earn a profit from my endeavors.

In those days, the typical patient that came to me seemed to be retired CEOs with a science background. I think that a CEO thinks differently about the world. The buck stops with them and they take in the information, carefully weigh it, and then can change the course of the ship if they need to. Engineers also have the tendency to ignore emotional or religious overtones and are very simple and causal in their reasoning.

In 2009, the Nobel Prize was awarded for the discovery of telomerase and the subsequent media coverage and legitimacy infused my practice with the hope it would need to become sustainable. More people began to show interest and I was being interviewed for TV news reports. My two-year project of getting my graphic novel completed was nearing an end and I dedicated myself to getting the word out about TA-65.

To do this, I learned how to host a live webinar, edit videos, and post them to YouTube and iTunes as podcasts. Interest from my blog postings began to grow my opt-in email list. I began to develop a fan base of patients and other freethinking people interested in slowing aging.

As we will discuss in the following chapter, many of my patients began to report amazing results. As a scientist, I have to be skeptical and consider the placebo effect and potential bias. However, when three separate people came forward with a similar report, I would plan a webinar. This pattern emerged for topics from hypertension, exercise, cancer, depression, and many others.

Since my YouTube channel's founding in September of 2010, I have produced 80 videos with 45 of them being live webinars lasting up to an hour. I have had over 120,000 views on YouTube and the number continues to grow rapidly. Each of these labors of love took between 20 and 40 hours to research, write, host, and edit but the experience I gained was invaluable. I learned so much about subjects that I otherwise wouldn't have understood. Doing the research and organizing my thoughts allowed me to develop my theories. Importantly, I also developed the voice that I would need to care for my patients, lecture to other physicians, and write this book.

TA-65 began at a dosage of 10mg when pioneers began using the technology in 2007. Caution over possible unforeseen effects proved unwarranted so everyone on the Patton Protocol was increased to 25mg, then in another 6 months to 50mg, then to 100mg. There simply were no reported side effects. They were not reporting diseases or cancer-- people were reporting anecdotal improvements that would become the subject of my many webinars.

In my experience, most people initially believe the TA-65 is helping, but their faith wanes. Only by stopping and restarting a few times can they fully appreciate the benefits.

After the initial gains in their quality of living, TA-65 users don't really see or feel much. That is a good thing because anything that alters mood or the mind is addictive and creates tolerance and withdrawal. Most people feel holistically better and they soon sleep better, eat better, exercise, and do other healthy habits that further enhance their health. I call this the "upward spiral."

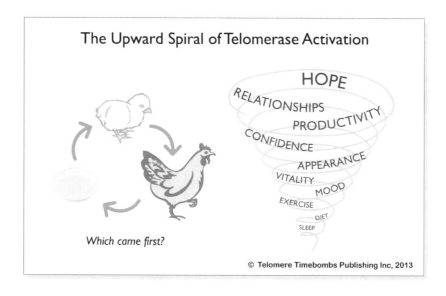

Holistic wellness: "It's not one thing, it's everything"

With the "upward spiral" and the ongoing expense, most clients experience "attribution fatigue." That is to say, they take credit for their improvements and say "I've always looked young for my age" and "I'm doing a lot of things" so they do not think to attribute their better health and wellbeing to the TA-65, per se.

That said, the majority of new patient growth appears to come from word of mouth referrals. Usually, a patient doesn't really become a "true believer" until stopping and restarting the TA-65 two or more times. I find that people think about their health like they think about the weather. They get used to it, take it for granted, and only talk about it when it's bad.

Restarting TA-65 after a break is like getting off a plane in a tropical airport. While settled into your winter vacation destination, you don't notice how nice it is. But if you leave and then come back, you can more fully appreciate the heat, humidity, and your mood is different as you walk down the jetway in Cancun versus boarding in Chicago O'Hare.

Another interesting phenomenon that often occurs at about four months or seven months of usage is that a patient's appearance can be noted as changed. While not noticeable to themselves or the people who see them on a daily basis, friends and acquaintances that rarely see them are often stunned at the more youthful appearances they present.

There are probably dozens of factors that people use to determine age. From posture, voice, diction, wrinkles, mood, odor...the list is long. Typically, my patients are asked why they look younger and often are accused of having procedures. They typically make note of it but say to themselves "I'm doing a lot of things and besides, I don't notice anything."

So where are we currently in the TA-65 story? There have been tens of thousands of people who have taken it without untoward effects (and no increases in cancer noted). There are over 600 doctors trained to provide it and the number increases daily. Is this the "fountain of youth" in a tiny capsule? I believe the answer is yes.

People have been taking TA-65 since the 2005 trial, with no significant adverse reactions reported. I firmly believe that TA-65 is safe and effective. I take it daily and have given it to my own children. So why mess with success? Would you drink a substance that was touted as artificial water? There are countless examples of pharmaceutical companies tweaking perfectly good drugs for a profit and ending up with something that has unforeseen side effects down the line.

That is not to say that the price won't come down or that another company won't bring to market another telomerase activator. But based upon my understanding of the safety, gene activation profile, and efficacy of this one, I'm not planning to try a different telomerase activator.

And just why do I think TA-65 works so well? That is the subject of the next chapter. Thanks for keeping an open mind and now, you can go and do research to verify that what I've told you is not just a story. You can start with the research shown below.

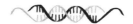

Studies Pertaining to TA

Fauce et al in *The Journal of Immunology* (2008): A telomerase activator discovered by the Geron Corporation was shown, via telomerase reverse transcription, to help especially HIV-infected T-cells to function, reproduce, and protect themselves better.

Harley et al in *Rejuvenation Research* (2011): Harley et al looked at the early Patton Protocol patients taking TA-65 and found that after starting a TA program, the percentage of burned-out CD28 negative cells fell dramatically, especially if the person was CMV infected. In addition, the percentage of cells with short telomeres (defined here as <4000 base pairs) decreased after TA-65 ingestion.

Bernardes de Jesus et al in *The Aging Cell* (2011): TA-65 was given to mice engineered to age because of a half-gene dosage of TERC. Via telomerase action, the average telomere length increased and the percent of critically-shortened telomeres decreased. Associated findings were more youthful glucose tolerance, better skin, less osteoporosis, and no increased cancer incidence.

Molgora et al in *Cells* (2013): Independent verification that TA-65 and not another alleged telomerase activator increased T-cell proliferation by increasing telomerase activity.

Professor Henry Jones: *Elsa never really believed in the grail. She thought she'd found a prize.*

Indiana Jones: *And what did you find, Dad?*

Professor Henry Jones: *Me? Illumination.*

—Indiana Jones and the Last Crusade — (Paramount Pictures, 1989)

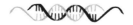

9

TELOMERASE ACTIVATION MEDICINE

We'll begin
With a spin
Traveling in
The world of my creation
What we'll see
Will defy
Explanation

If you want to view paradise
Simply look around and view it
Anything you want to, do it
Wanta change the world?
There's nothing
To it

Willie Wonka. Willie Wonka & the Chocolate Factory
(Warner Bros., 1971)

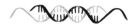

This long chapter is really a book within this book. Think of it as a little leather-bound journal, like something a 19th century naturalist or 20th century anthropologist would sketch and write in. It is all about anecdotes and patterns that I have noted from many years of clinical experience with real patients taking a telomerase activator. We are pioneers who have used this new but most ancient of technologies to naturally reverse aging and improve health by tapping into the abundance of life itself. I call what I have been practicing, telomerase activation medicine.

I have four big goals for this chapter:

1) discuss what evidence-based medicine is;
2) provide my theories on the four mechanisms of how telomerase activation may be helping;
3) describe the "typical" effects of telomerase activation; and
4) present some amazing cases of clinical improvement after taking a telomerase activator.

The dilemma for this chapter is the following: you will read some incredible true stories and it is up to you to decide whether it is faith healing, the placebo effect, or something more.

The image you should have is one of me, sitting countless hours, following up with patients on the phone, answering emails, and researching on the internet to produce over 80 videos, and give lectures across the country. Like you, I am appropriately skeptical of what I hear from my patients because it often does verge on the realm of "praise God!" faith healing at times. When one of my patients tells me something has improved, I don't think much of it, when two tell me, I take note, but when the third person comes forward, I generally do a live webinar on the subject.

When people have improvements after taking a telomerase activator, is it all imagined? Just to be clear, the placebo effect is real and that is because the mind is part of the body and the body is able to heal itself quite extensively. Also, there is a lot of what statisticians call "bias" in the recollection and attribution of effects that may not be causally related to an intervention. But if TA-65 really does nothing, I must be the most amazing mesmerist to have ever walked the face of the earth.

If my patients and I are conjuring up real, measurable objective changes for the better, it shouldn't much matter whether it is a placebo effect or not. When my friend's dad's brain cancer goes away or a 114-year-old woman sprouts black hairs, it is strictly anecdotal, I know. But the fact is that the science is sound, my theories are logical, and the research supports telomere erosion is related to both brain cancer and hair color. Besides, nobody is being paid to make stuff up. On the contrary, all my patients are paying customers and they are looking for a reason to disbelieve because of the expense.

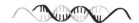

Evidence-based Medicine

Overall, we are still in Schopenhauer's "ignore" stage but if any of my medical colleagues would deign to look at "telomerase activation medicine," they would strongly object based on a sort of kneejerk cry for "evidence-based medicine." But prejudice means pre-judging and skeptics usually won't even review the peer-reviewed studies of TA-65 that I cite to them.

The truth of the matter is that most people are afraid to think for themselves unless they are given permission to do so. This is especially true when it comes to something they strongly yet secretly desire to be true.

The premise of this cult of evidence-based medicine that developed out of epidemiology is that it is better to practice medicine based upon studies that have been published and peer-reviewed whenever possible. That sounds very good and in fact, IS very good. However, conclusions are prone to errors from the underlying explanatory model, study design, data, investigator integrity and bias.

When making decisions on behalf of patients, there are four levels of evidence quality recognized. They are listed here from soundest to weakest:

Level I: evidence from at least one properly designed randomized control trial (which is not to say that multiple studies can't contradict each other because they often do.)

Level II-1: evidence from well-designed trials without randomization. For example, you couldn't blindly randomize people for exercise as an intervention because they would be aware that they were participating in exercise.

Level II-2: evidence from case-control studies or cohort studies. This would be like going through the records of women who required blood transfusions in labor and seeing if certain practices were associated with that outcome.

Level II-3: evidence from time series such as following a cohort of nurses over decades and reporting patterns that emerge from the data.

Level III: anecdotal evidence or opinions of experts. But note well that in the gladiatorial sport of hand waving, speculation, and theorizing, I am on equal footing with even the most august of professors and Nobel Prize winners.

Anecdotes are not scientific proof. However, consider that many fields of human endeavors are anecdotally-based: criminal law, anthropology, sports recruiting, social hierarchy, online restaurant recommendations, and on and on.

I would venture to say there are actually almost no decisions we make that are not anecdotally-based or simply chosen on the basis of obedience to conventional wisdom, word of mouth, or our intuition. Have you read the latest randomized controlled trials on your toothpaste, laundry detergent, voting record, or choice of friends? We simply go by intuition, which is a dynamic system of pattern recognition based upon emotions, knowledge, wisdom, probability, and game theory.

The last and most important disclaimer involves what we can and can't say about causation. TA-65 is not a drug. It is classified as a plant-derived nutraceutical. This means that it comes from a plant which has been ingested safely as a potentially beneficial herb and that no claims of disease prevention and treatment can be made about its use.

TA-65 is not, nor will it ever be FDA-approved to treat any disease because of reasons we will explore in Chapter 10: "The Medical-industrial complex." Since aging is not a disease by standard definitions, I can and do assert that it can reverse the signs and symptoms of aging.

But me thinks I doth disclaim too much. Just don't try to use your built-in "BS detector" while you are ensconced in the reading of this chapter because it will be like some annoying kid shouting out his guesses about a magician's sleight of hand at a children's party. Just enjoy the show for now. You can look up my YouTube videos and use your intuition to judge whether the patients' stories are believable or not. That is not only your right, it is your moral obligation.

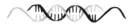

Four possible modes of improvement while taking a TA

The main effect of taking a nutraceutical telomerase activator is a temporary increase in the transcription of the telomerase micromachines, thereby allowing for more telomerase activity to take place in that cell. As we discussed in Chapter 4: "Telomerase," only the stem cells can produce telomerase. Differentiated, non-stem cells have epigenetic changes that prevent the transcription and expression of their copies of the telomerase enzyme. Telomerase activity in stem cells is "always on" but appears to increase up to 300% while the telomerase activation, or enhancement, is transiently stimulated by an ingested TA. This statement is based on proprietary, unpublished data belonging to the T.A. Sciences Corporation and validated by Molgora et al in *Cells* (2013).

As a result of this action, I believe changes arising from telomerase activation have at least four distinct mechanisms of action: 1) prevention; 2) faster replication; 3) stochastic changes; and 4) apoptosis.

Interestingly, there also exist so-called "non-canonical" or non-reverse transcriptase-related functions of telomerase that we will not explore here.

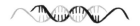

The First TA Mechanism (Prevention through Lengthening)

The first possible TA mechanism is that of damage prevention. It is the most obvious because it states that when telomerase activity increases, telomeres grow longer. Longer telomeres mean that the cell's date with destiny, or its chromosomal damage from erosion, is postponed. But consider that if the stem cells are already damaged, this could be viewed as a bad thing because perhaps the already damaged stem cell you would want to replace would soon have continued to damage itself right out of existence.

As with car maintenance, prevention earlier is more effective. Just like it is better to change the oil in your Ferrari every three thousand miles rather than every 40,000, it will probably prove more prudent and cost-effective to take a telomerase activator in your 20's rather than your 60's.

As we discussed in Chapter 6: "Telomere erosion in disease," the risk for all cancers increases with telomere erosion. Active prevention of that erosion may someday be shown to play a role in delaying the development of cancers everywhere.

Is this preventative effect measurable? Yes! In the case of one 79 year-old patient, the median telomere length increased from 4100 base pairs to 5400 after two years of ingesting a telomerase activator. There are alternative hypotheses for why this happened, but because it occurred in the presence of amazing clinical improvements, we must also consider the possibility that the TA helped. Evidence-based medicine might cast derision upon this result but I know he sleeps better at night knowing he has gained 13 years of leukocyte telomere length since he began at the age of 77!

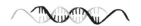

The Second TA Mechanism: Accelerated Copying

Because the rate-limiting step of a stem cell division is probably copying the 6 gigabytes of DNA information, anything that speeds up the process will help cells copy faster. As we know, there is always a need for ongoing telomerase activity because without that, stem cell telomeres would shorten and they would become bad master copies.

Accelerated copying is a great explanation for two interesting phenomena resulting from taking a telomerase activator: more restful sleep and faster healing. Because sleep is both physical repair and the synthesis of new brain cells, a more efficient and rapid stem cell copying would explain why the sleep is often qualitatively different in the majority of patients who take TA before sleep. The more rapid and efficient stem cell copying also might explain enhanced healing from skin wounds and exercise soreness.

These effects are immediate and real-time and I have advised people that if they can't afford TA daily, then take it like aspirin. In other words, save it for nights when you are stressed and apt to sleep poorly, or after you have been injured, out partying, or overdone it with exercising. If you take TA before sleep tonight, the dreams and sleeping will be better. If you don't take it tomorrow night, they will be unchanged unless stochastic effects are still in play. This indicates the benefit is real-time and probably a result of increase efficiency of cell replication.

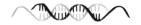

The Third TA Mechanism: Stochastics

The third way I believe TA works is, for want of a better word, is stochastically. Stochastics is a term used very differently by many different fields. Stochastically is meant to indicate that the system is complex and not deterministic. In other words, you can't predict what will happen because there are so many probabilistic factors and emergent properties. What I really mean to say is something more like "enhancement of the fittest."

As we will discuss with mood, energy, and libido, the effects can wax stronger after a few days, and after stopping a TA, the effects can also wane after a few days to weeks. Because all stem cells are benefitting, it stands to reason that the ones that are younger and healthier will benefit more, thereby giving the niche, the organ, the functioning, and the person a boost. Think of it like giving bicycles to people to finish a foot race. Everyone benefits but the 20-year-old benefits more than the 80-year-old because he pedals faster for longer.

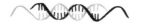

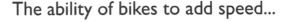
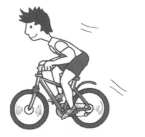
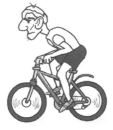
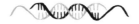

The ability of bikes to add speed...

Depends on the quality of the athelete

© Telomere Timebombs Publishing Inc, 2013

Improved telomerase can affect cells differently

It isn't "survival of the fittest" because the stronger and weaker queen bees still coexist. It's just that the stronger queen makes more copies of her smarter and better-looking kids so they are all are over-represented for extra days to weeks while taking a TA. Other good examples of stochastic advantage at work would be aerobic performance, skin appearance, rate of nail growth.

The Fourth TA Mechanism: Apoptosis
When the telomeres become critically-short and no longer serve their capping function, the DNA breakage repair team comes in and attaches that end of the chromosome to somewhere it doesn't belong (discussed in Chapter 3: "What is a telomere?"). It's like trying to divide a deck of cards into two piles of 26 black

and 26 red cards when the Queen of Hearts and the Queen of Spades are glued together.

Recall that when the chromosomes line up, the p53 enzyme, the watchmen of the genome, can receive a signal indicating the chromosomal distribution will be uneven. In that instance, p53 starts the suicide program by causing the hundreds of mitochondria to leak out their battery acid and melt the cell from inside like the Wicked Witch of the East after being doused by water.

As cited in the previous chapter, experiments have shown that TA-65 given to mice will decrease the percentage of critically-short telomeres and that giving TA-65 will cause the percentage of senescent or burned out T-cells to decrease. It is clear to me that somehow, telomerase activation enables more efficient apoptosis although the exact mechanism remains to be elucidated.

I believe it's like having a stripped Philips-head screw as the last thing you need to disassemble a broken machine. Perhaps adding telomeres allows the "handling" of the chromosomes to occur like restoring the grooves on the head of the screw.

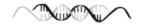

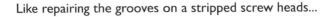

Like repairing the grooves on a stripped screw heads...

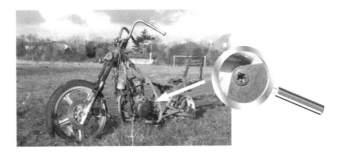

Telomerase activation permits stem cell self-destruction to finally occur

© Telomere Timebombs Publishing Inc, 2013

TA appears to facilitate apoptosis

The apoptosis of damaged stem cells may be producing the most interesting changes we see, such as hair repigmentation, weight loss, improvement of symptoms of disease, and resolution of chronic degenerative changes.

After stopping a TA, patients might lament a return to the preexisting quality of sleep, mood, and fatigue. However, there are often permanent improvements because of the apoptotic changes that can result. Interestingly, even if the death of the stem cell queen bee happens immediately, it may take four or seven months for the effects to manifest because the descendants of the dead queen have to burn through their telomeres. I don't know why four and seven months are clinically important but it must have something to do with the Hayflick limit in those organs.

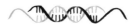

Typical Effects of Taking a TA

This is the fun part of this chapter but I should warn you by saying that everyone is different. Just as a car with 50,000 miles that has never been serviced won't have the same exact issues as another one driven under different conditions in a different climate, so no two TA patients respond the same.

Also, changes can be immediate, or they can take time to manifest, as I just mentioned. It's kind of like spelunking, which is a term for cave exploring. Sometimes, you find a hidden passage out of the cave, but more likely, you have to walk back out and up just as far as it took to go in and down to your current location. In other words, you don't get old overnight and so, you don't get younger overnight.

Contrary to the package insert guidelines for the TA-65 product, I generally, but not always, recommend that my patients take the TA before sleep, or within fourteen hours of planned awakening. I do that because I believe that the most active time of repair and cell replication is during sleep. Just like you don't repair a highway during rush hour, the body spends most of the day in active and catabolic, or destructive work.

During sleep, growth hormone, one of the anabolic (growth-promoting) hormones peaks during the first two deep sleep cycles of the night. In the third and subsequent cycles, the critical neurogenesis (new brain cell creation) that is involved in dreaming and the defragmentation of the mind takes place.

Around 90% of patients appear to have qualitative changes in their sleep, even at low doses of a telomerase activator. Although it would seem to be quite subjective, one of the most sensitive and specific alterations is that dreaming becomes more vivid. The content is more emotionally-charged, colorful, references things buried deep in the past, and is generally more "fun." If you go to bed anxious and in a scarcity mindset, however, the dreams can be very unpleasant nightmares although as a saving grace, they often point to "solutions" or feature you as more active protagonist.

A mental state is called a quale (plural: qualia) and it is a philosophical concept to describe our subjective experience of something, or the way things seem to us. For example, it's like the taste of wine, receiving a standing ovation, or the way your experience a scene in a dream. Well, the qualia experienced in your dreams become so vivid that often people report being confused about whether something happened in waking life or whether it occurred in their dream. Thankfully, they always seem to figure it out later although the experience immediately upon awakening can be very odd.

Awakening is another interesting thing. Because sleep occurs in cycles, the brainstem has to awaken you each time and for some reason, this happens with the force of a dolphin jumping for a smelt, rather than a bubble rising in a glass of sparkling water.

Because I warn my patients that they may wake up at 3AM feeling like it's 8AM, they don't worry and are back to sleep in seconds. If they act like a flying fish rather than a dolphin, they might get up and check email. Big mistake. We still need a good four cycles (6 hours) to restore mind and body and the mind will immediately go back into sleep if you let it.

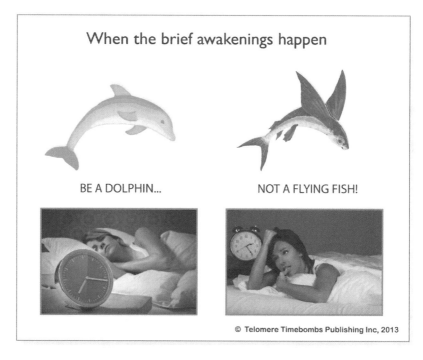

When the brief awakenings happen

BE A DOLPHIN...

NOT A FLYING FISH!

© Telomere Timebombs Publishing Inc, 2013

**Being wide-awake after every 90-minute
sleep cycle can occur on TA**

With time, the brief awakenings that occur between sleep cycles tend to happen less noticeably, then less frequently, then not at all. During times of higher anxiety or life force, these brief awakening can recur however, and sometimes require a modification of TA dosing.

Some people say they don't dream. They actually do. But older people or those with significant neurological injury do not recall dreaming well, possibly because it just isn't very vivid. Other neurologically intact people seem to repress their recollection of dreams as a general policy of the superego, if you will. But even older, non-dreamers can resume dream recollection in my experience although it usually takes seven to thirteen months to manifest.

Another interesting phenomenon related to sleep is the entrainment of the circadian rhythm. Circadian rhythm is your internal clock and it gets cleaned, if you will. This means people tend to get sleepy the exact same time each day. Also, the drowsiness comes in waves of six hours generally. I tend to get sleepy at noon, 6 PM, and midnight. Also, I have found that taking TA helps people overcome jet lag very well.

Finally, daytime drowsiness is not uncommon in the first two weeks. It is as though you hit Control-Alt-Delete or the old Microsoft "Blue screen of death" comes up and you simply need to shut down. I believe this is the consciousness of the body, along with the circadian rhythm, asking you for 'down time' to repair. A fifteen-minute catnap is often enough to take care of it in most cases.

For more information on sleep, dreams and circadian rhythms, see Podcasts 9, 35 and 39 respectively on my YouTube channel, "*drpark65.*"

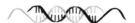

For a variety of possible reasons, many people experience improved mood by the fourth day of TA ingestion. Certainly the improved sleep is contributing, as is the optimism of starting a new supplement. But I believe there may be a stochastic and apoptotic element as well. It is as though the neurotransmitters are just more charged and the psyche is more grounded. Of note, this sense of wellbeing is not euphoria per se, and there is never any 'come down.' Often people note that many things that used to annoy them don't seem to bother them as much anymore. I believe that this is not a chemical effect but rather a stochastic, cellular effect; the cells are functioning better so it is sustainable.

I want to emphasize that taking a pure TA shouldn't have psychotropic actions such as euphoria or psychomotor acceleration (the feeling from caffeine or stimulants). People don't feel any different, which is good. With changes in mood would come tolerance (needing increasing doses to feel the same 'high'), dependence (a craving for the "fix"), and withdrawal symptoms (the bad feeling or "dysphoria" that comes from abstinence). You can take twelve capsules one night and none the next and it won't change your mood or mental functioning directly.

Within the first two weeks, many people experience a tightening of the skin and their nails begin to grow rapidly. Hair changes are variable but often the hair begins to grow faster. The keratin-producing stem cells for the hair, skin, and nails seem to "kick it up a notch."

This stands to reason because recall that dyskeratosis congenita is a failure of telomerase activity so increasing the activity would tend to reverse the symptoms of aging hair, skin and nails.

If you chart the rate of adult human nail growth, it declines after age 25. Aging has begun to set in by our mid 20s and the decline, which I believe is the result of accumulation of damage in stem cells, will take its toll on other youthful traits such as libido, athletic performance, and mental acuity.

Another incredibly subjective indication, but one with a high positive predictive value, is the "unsolicited compliment sign." I would say that 7 out of 10 patients begin receiving multiple unsolicited remarks about their improved and more youthful appearance by seven months. Interestingly, the majority of those patients don't think it is related to taking a TA because they are "doing a lot of things." And they invariably boast they've always looked young for their age. These are usually the patients who are most alarmed when the telomere measurement fails to bolster their youthful self-image.

This reluctant attribution of improvement to TA usage may come from a fear of becoming aesthetically dependent on TA. It also comes from what I like to call the "upward spiral," the little-known sibling of the downward spiral, and speaks to panacea-like changes that telomerase activation can play in all stem cell types.

Some more scientifically inclined patients intentionally try keeping as much constant routine and habits as possible so as to be more objective about changes on TA. But more often, the upward spiral resulting from multiple changes in behavior is evident: patients start meditating, going vegetarian, doing more exercise, and engaging more positively with their lives. The upward spiral isn't just one thing, it's everything. Sure, exercise alone could account for many positive changes, but the TA helps people with their motivation, the ability to recover, and optimism to transform their lives on many fronts.

I recall a 53-year-old friend of mine who discontinued taking TA after three months, declaring that he didn't need it because of the yoga he was doing. That seemed plausible so I asked "how long have you been doing yoga?" He replied that he hadn't done yoga for the last nine years because of back pain but since the TA, he had resumed it without any problem.

That reminds me of a Vespa Scooter I had in college and a power-lifter client. I used to have a scooter with a slippery kick-starter. If the starter was slipping, I would have to push the thing, running at its side, then pop it out of neutral into second gear to get started. And then we were roaring along without any problem. The same principle was at work with my 41-year-old client who came to me very thin and weak. After taking TA-65, he began to compete and win as a competitive power lifter against twenty-somethings. He stopped taking the TA after 6 months but the improvements continued. Why? His Vespa was running and he was in an exercise-aided upward spiral.

Increased libido is an interesting change that relates to mood, hormone levels, body self-image, and interpersonal chemistry. Men often report improved erectile function, and both men and women report improved libido. I'll never forget what one of my 52-year-old patients noted at her one-year follow-up on TA-65. Her breast size had gone from an "A" to a "B" cup and she thought it was odd that she hadn't had a fight with her husband for the preceding six months. Any husbands reading that last sentence might want to put down the book and call my office right now.

If these vignettes interest you, there are many more remarkable anecdotes that I don't have time to explore here. It's 1.2 days' worth of video content, after all. If you are interested in learning more, I would urge you to go to my website at www.rechargebiomedical.com.

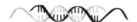

The Love Child

Nina was a 41-year-old clinical psychologist, only 96 pounds, and a yoga instructor who had not menstruated for two years. When she married in her early 30s, she underwent assisted reproduction with ovarian hyperstimulation and despite the anguish, time, and expense had only an early miscarriage to show for it. Nina had given up on having children long ago and although it threatened to break them up some years earlier, she and her older, childless husband had reconciled themselves that it was never meant to be.

Not surprisingly, trying to "shock and awe" her fertility "disease" into submission with a medical assault failed. There are many things that need to go right to take home a healthy baby. First, you need good sperm and young, intact eggs that haven't suffered nondisjunction, which as will you recall from Chapter 3: "What is a telomere?" is uneven chromosomal separation. Recall that nondisjunction occurs in all our aging stem cells when the telomeres become critically-shortened but when it occurs in the ovarian stem cells, conditions like Down's Syndrome can occur.

Secondly, you need to ovulate. Ovulation is inhibited by aging of ovarian stem cells, stress, and low body fat. Third, you need to have sexual relations at the exact right time, and frequency helps with that. Fourth, you need to implant, grow, and maintain the fertilized egg, which in the case of high anxiety and cortisol levels can be problematic.

While on vacation, Nina commented to her mother that she was having breast enlargement and tenderness. Having previously suffered severe nausea during pregnancy, she knew that couldn't be the reason and was worried it could be cancer. Her mother insisted she take a pregnancy test anyway to which she laughed and told her she hadn't had a period for years. But come to think of it, she had been having sexual relations with her husband lately after having little to no interest for years.

You could have knocked her over with a feather when the result came back positive. Nine months later, she had a beautiful and healthy baby although her pregnancy was very rocky due to nausea, high blood pressure, and stress that manifested soon after stopping TA-65.

Is TA-65 safe during pregnancy? I don't know. I can say that the cells are bathing in telomerase activity because they are very stem-like during the growth of the fetus. Consider also that from conception to birth you and I burned through a third of our endowment, from 15,000 to 10,000 base pairs. So it is entirely possible that six weeks of unusually increased telomerase activity slowed the attrition and that little one was born with an endowment of 11,000, or an extra decade of life expectancy. What we can say is that despite coming from a 41-year-old egg and receiving TA-65 during the critical formation of his organs, there were no birth defects in this happy lovechild of rekindled midlife passion.

Why did this occur? Well, this is not an FDA-approved statement but I would guess that her mood and energy improved, her feelings of intimacy and sexiness improved, her anti-ovulatory stress dropped, and that her eggs were rescued to ovulate by telomerase activation. During her pregnancy, she suffered horrible anxiety and high blood pressure and we hope that didn't affect the child. But when her post-partum depression became unbearable off the TA-65, she resumed taking it and her mood immediately improved. Now, at age 43, she is excited about having even more children.

Regarding rescue stimulation of ovulation that can occur, I have had several patients taking TA-65 resume menstruating long after menopause; up to 13 years after in the case of a 63-year-old although it generally doesn't last many months. It is kind of like finding a gallon of gas in your trunk. Bleeding post-menopausally can be a sign of uterine cancer so it shouldn't be ignored and just assumed to be ovulation. But if the patient has monthly bleeding, no cancer on her uterine biopsy, premenstrual symptoms like moodiness, breast tenderness, and food cravings, and a low FSH, or follicle stimulating hormone (which is the signal from the brain to the ovaries), that would all strongly suggest a resumption of menstruation.

For more information on female fertility, see Podcast 41 on my YouTube channel, *"drpark65."*

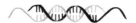

Back to Life after Praying for Death

Four years ago, Margarete was stopped at a traffic light. Her mind wandered as she though how lucky she was. Fifty-six years old, comfortable, successful on her own terms, athletic, and simply the master of her domain. She thought to herself "life just doesn't get any better than this."

Speeding towards her stationary bumper was an anxious woman, rechecking her email to make sure she was really reading what she was reading. "It just doesn't get any worse than this," she thought to herself.

It would turn out that Margarete was spot on, but the lady who rear-ended her was wrong. Life was about to get a lot worse for both of them.

Margarete's pelvis was shattered as were four out of five of her lumbar vertebrae. The remaining backbones were all fractured to varying degrees.

After the accident, she felt a constant, belt-like pain around her chest. Her short-term memory was shot. But the worst was to come months later when an unrecognized fractured rib punctured her stomach like a stiletto knife. This caused massive internal organ damage that almost killed her and required removal of her stomach.

The absence of her stomach to sterilize food led to an overgrowth of an opportunistic bacterium species called *Clostridium difficile*. The foul-smelling, painful diarrhea is so virulent that it would have easily overwhelmed and killed her if not for continuous courses of powerful antibiotics.

The times she had tried to go off of the antibiotics, the Clostridial diarrhea would return with a vengeance and she knew there would never be any hope for stopping the dangerous medications.

Worst of all was the chronic pain of her low back and the belt-like pain around her chest. This required round-the-clock use of powerful narcotics to even maintain consciousness. She couldn't sleep restfully and for 23 hours a day, her psyche was constantly ravaged by the unbearable pain.

She kept from her family her passionate longing to die. Her quality of life could only improve if she were dead, she reasoned. The will power it took to fight the constant pain, stave off the infectious diarrhea, and try to get some rest was indescribably exhausting. She kept her hope alive only with morbid anticipation of "slipping the surly bonds of Earth," as the poet and aviator John Magee described in his poem "High Flight."

Immediately after starting TA-65, Margarete quickly began to improve. Her mood, sleep, and pain all began to transform back to modes from years ago when there were cycles, pleasures, and respites. These began to return, in contrast to the constant white noise din of suffering that constituted her existential hell of a life since the accident and rupture of her stomach.

Within one month she attempted and succeeded in stopping oral antibiotics and for the first time, the diarrhea did not recur. Better still, she was sleeping ten hours a night and was no longer requiring round-the-clock narcotics to stay sane.

What was the change that occurred? You can watch my podcasts on back pain, constipation and addictions to learn more. Suffice it to say that Margarete was convinced the changes occurred as a direct result of taking TA-65.

As she put it, "before TA-65, I had no hope for living. I wanted to die. Now, I can honestly say that I have hope. The TA-65 gave me my life back."

To hear more about Margarete's story, watch Podcast 45 about "constipation" on my YouTube channel, *"drpark65."*

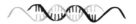

Brain Cancer Cured by the Anti-placebo Effect?
Mr. Lee (not his real name) is a 67 year-old man without brain cancer. That bears mentioning because at age 62, he had a high-grade oligodendroglioma that was encompassing half his brain.

Having already lived through my father's horrible decline on standard treatment, I was eager to help my friend's father by suggesting he try TA-65. I had recently heard about Walt, whose wife's brain cancer disappeared after only one month of taking the telomerase activator, despite having failed all other therapies. For more info on brain cancer, please see Podcast 29 on YouTube.

Because it was so extensive, Mr. Lee's tumor was inoperable and he received whole brain radiation, followed by oral chemotherapy with Temodar®, a standard treatment that causes DNA damage in all cells. This was done with the hopes that rapidly reproducing cells will be more damaged than friendly ones. Unfortunately, the brain tumor continued to grow while he was on Temodar.

Mr. Lee then took Avastin®, an experimental antibody that blocks new blood vessel formation, despite still not being FDA-approved for this indication at the time of this writing in mid-2013. The tumor continued to grow on Avastin.

The doctors added Carboplatin, another DNA-mutating chemotherapy agent, and the tumor growth slowed briefly but it soon resumed again. This prompted the resumption of Temodar even though the tumor had previously grown while taking it. Doctors don't like sitting back and doing nothing and they don't trust the body to rid itself of the disease.

My friend and I, against the wishes of all his family members, finally persuaded Mr. Lee to try TA-65 in February of 2011; he took it for a year.

Immediately after starting the TA, he called to complain about a side effect: allergies. He was livid that the March pollen was making him sneeze and causing congestion. It seems that for the previous three years, his lifelong allergies were gone, probably due to immune suppression from cancer and chemotherapy.

I explained that this was probably a good sign that meant his immune system was recovering. But he remained upset about sneezing and having to buy Claritin® and tissues.

For whatever reason, two years after taking TA-65, and six years after being diagnosed with inoperable brain cancer that had grown to cover half his brain despite all the best medicines insurance money could buy, there is no trace of his brain cancer on MRI.

Is there an "anti-placebo" effect? Mr. Lee scoffs at the possibility that TA-65 could have helped him despite understanding the tumor was overwhelming him prior to starting it. His physicians, as with Walt's wife, held case conferences to marvel at the apparent cure, but Mr. Lee won't tell them about the TA-65 because he is afraid of losing his health insurance. As we will discuss in the next chapter, that fear looms over many people in this medical-industrial dystopia of high-priced, rationed yet irrational disease maintenance misbranded as health care or health maintenance.

To say that eradication of an extensive, high-grade brain cancer is not common is like saying "you just don't see a lot of unicorns these days." TA-65 is not a treatment for brain cancer or FDA-approved to treat any disease. That said, I am hoping someone will come forth and do a randomized-controlled trial testing this exciting possible breakthrough. I have written to UCSF where the doctors treated Walt's wife, and put a challenge at the end of my video. So what could be the possible mechanism of this? I believe it would be apoptosis of the cancer stem cells as discussed in Chapters 3 and 5.

As mentioned, we are still in Schopenhauer's "ignore" phase so I can't even get someone to make fun of me. I can't even get my friend, a brain surgeon who takes TA-65 daily, to watch my video on brain cancer! Why not? The next chapter will explore the crypto-fascist quasi-religious system we sometimes call Western allopathic medicine, or what I like to call the "Medical-industrial complex." By the way, I'm not endorsing osteopathy, homeopathy or naturopathy. I'm just letting you know that allopathic is a slightly pejorative term those outsiders use for us mainstream medical docs.

And that, my friends, concludes my brief tour of the Wonka Chocolate Factory of telomerase activation medicine. You may now reengage your healthy skepticism and if you so desire, verify what I have told you by watching my videos and by doing your own due diligence.

The stories, interpretations, and extrapolations that produced this chapter may someday prove to be wrong, but I wouldn't have written them down if I thought so.

Remember how I told you my favorite screenplay was the one that I wrote about the 4th century philosopher and civil rights martyr Hypatia? Here is one of her quotes that I will wear as a fig leaf if I am tarred, feathered, and run out of town on the proverbial rail for sharing my clinical experiences with you:

> *"Reserve your right to think, for even to think wrongly is better than not to think at all."*

> — Hypatia (4th century philosopher)

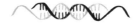

10

THE MEDICAL-INDUSTRIAL COMPLEX

There is a war between the rich and poor,

A war between the man and the woman.

There is a war between the ones who say there is a war
And the ones who say there isn't.

Why don't you come on back to the war, that's right, get in it,
Why don't you come on back to the war, it's just beginning.

— Leonard Cohen, "There is a war"

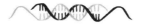

The purpose of this chapter is to vent about what I believe is wrong with the world today. My soap box, please. A warning: if you feel a strong congenital compulsion to deny that our leaders in academia, commerce, and government have anything but the most noble intentions, then please skip this chapter. It will anger you. Seriously, go to Chapter 11: "The Future" right now! Do not pass "Go" and don't collect my two cents either.

If you are still reading, let me start by saying that I believe the recurring dilemma of any mindful person is deciding how much responsibility to defer to others when it comes to learning the truth. The images that we will work with are a silver-haired warrior/king and a silver and black-haired merry prankster.

From sinner to saint, no one gets out of here alive. We all know what will happen as we age and it isn't pretty. I haven't exaggerated or misled you and there have been tens of thousands who have safely tried telomerase activation and grown younger for it, so why wouldn't you consider trying something that is science-based, immediate in its effects, and is safe and effective?

That is not a rhetorical question, by the way. I believe the answer is that most people adhere to a blind faith in authority because they are lazy or need permission to think. My compulsion to ask "why" has disabused me of this faith in received wisdom and I will confess that I am prone to at least hearing out most conspiracy theories, which are sometimes marginalized versions of truth that threaten someone in power.

When you see a movie like "The Fugitive" (Warner Bros, 1993) in which Harrison Ford's character is framed for the murder of his own wife by some bad guys who want to get an unsafe drug approved, does your mind reel and say "Impossible!" Sadly, no.

From the "sinking" of the USS Maine as a pretext to start the Spanish-American War, to the fluoridation of the water supply (although I may be a bit early on this one), to the kids who were unjustly convicted after "confessing" to the Central Park "Wilding" Jogger rape, many wacko conspiracy theories eventually become rehabilitated into truth.

Americans are moral tightrope artists with a very big net below that we used to call Manifest Destiny but now bears the battleground title of "American exceptionalism." Why don't more people research and evaluate conspiracy theories? By analogy, would you want to read your mother and father's FBI files if someone told you they heard rumors they were a sex worker and a counterfeiter before you were born?

Our laziness and learned helplessness lets us hold onto the hope that our trappings of free speech, an arguably independent judiciary, and almost free press will safeguard the truth and preserve our liberties. Will it really? As Adolph Hitler allegedly said: "What good fortune for governments that the people do not think" (attribution unknown.)

There is and always has been a perpetual war, my friends, make no mistake. It is not Monsanto versus Greenpeace, or Fox News versus global warming enthusiasts. The true war is waged for the right to think freely. That war has always been waged by those few in power against each other, and against the masses who could prove dangerous if they were allowed to think something other than canonical versions of truth served up to them like cake from Marie Antoinette's ovens.

Modern Americans are a bit like the founding infants of Rome: Romulus and Remus. We are constantly being suckled by the she-wolf whose teats, ABC, CNN, ESPN, the AP, NPR, and MGM nourish us with the milk of programmed reality. The milk of the she-wolf, or "La Lupa," tells us that the bombs in the NFL Super Bowl are a matter of life and death, whereas unmanned drones falling from the sky in a far off land are a mere abstraction. The milk's narcotic urges us to delight in our celebrities' lovers and addictions but offers little guidance on how to cherish and master our own.

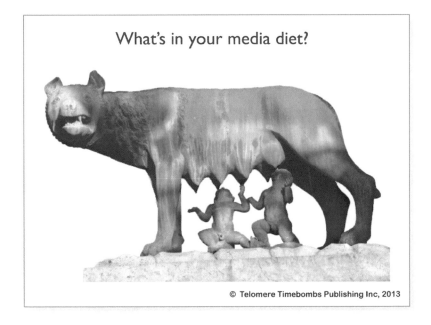

There are other types of nourishment out there

So what's my point in all this ranting? As The Beatles told us, "think for yourself." If everything you read here and watched on my website makes sense and is credible, read on.

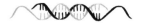

Holistic has Always Been Here

In the advance guard of this war are many people who are raising their consciousness about so-called alternative and complimentary, holistic or integrative medicine. And they are doing it the same way that I did: by surfing the internet, communicating with others, and reading until their beliefs came to mesh with the intuitive wisdom of knowing that life is abundant and good, not scarce and degenerate, as modern medicine would have it.

Without question, I believe that telomerase activation is the most disruptive and liberating new paradigm to come along since the Ninety-Five Theses of Martin Luther challenged the Catholic Church's monopoly on the truth and sparked the Protestant Reformation.

Your received values and beliefs about aging and health may be like the courtyard in the Turkish prison from *Midnight Express* (Casablanca Filmworks, 1978). We all are prisoners of a sort, choosing to walk clockwise around the pillar of authority, whether it's the FDA, academics, drug companies, doctors, or own limiting beliefs about how life was meant to be.

Speaking of doctors, when my patients ask me whether their own doctor will approve of taking a TA, I answer with 99% certainty, "No." Trying to get a mainstream doctor to accept the idea of reversing aging is like walking into Vatican City and proposing that they start worshiping a blue Hindu elephant god named Ganesha. Ain't gonna happen.

When my patients ask their personal physicians whether they could live to be 90 years old, the doctors reply, without any trace of irony, is "God, I hope not. You don't want to be 90." What a monstrous thing to say to a person. But it belies the macabre core beliefs of the medical profession and its ethos.

Sadly, I have come to realize that the irrefutable core value of my colleagues is hopelessness. We shouldn't swear to abide by the Hippocratic Oath; instead, we should be taking the Hypocrite's Oath. The dictum of "*primum non nocere*" (firstly, do no harm) could rightly be replaced with *"primum non spes providere"* or (firstly, don't give any hope).

We attended medical school, learned to treat patients, keep our minds and skills sharp, but we do harm patients all the time. And what's worse, we sleep soundly at night and wake up happy with the ghoul in the mirror and as long as we don't deviate from the mantra that life is hopeless and that the body is meant to decay. Standard, ineffective and harmful therapy inoculates us from malpractice concerns and low self-esteem, just as a drone strike launched from a destroyer means our government doesn't kill people on our behalf.

Forgive the off topic, slightly hysterical rant, but how did we go from a world where there was once outrage at the suggestion that a Russian president might have had a journalist and political detractor poisoned with radioactive sushi to now requiring laws to prohibit our government from droning U.S. citizens to death? How long before we are actually living in *The Matrix* (Warner Bros, 1999) or struggling in a world like that shown in *The Terminator* (Hemdale Film, 1984,) where "SKYNET," the self-aware machine god has usurped our humanity?

In the case of the greater world at large, who is creating this dystopian America? Surprising, there is a conspiracy but we are the greatest perpetrators of it upon ourselves. The false matrix of reality is generated when we allow someone else to decide what is acceptable and real on our behalf.

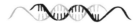

In the case of the Medical-industrial complex, who is to blame? Am I accusing someone of something? To paraphrase Émile Zola, *"Oui, J'accuse."* I accuse the modern physician of no longer being a healer but a line worker in a plant owned and operated by dark forces. We have relinquished the art of clinical medicine: to empathetically engage with the whole person, hear their story, understand their needs, and then earn their assent to therapy with all the courage, creativity and wisdom we can manifest.

My colleagues and I are being trained as disease management technicians who push newer and less effective drugs that beget new complications year after year until all natural systems fail or your Medicare supplemental insurance runs out of money. Wouldn't it be more cost effective to society to prevent all systems from failing by keeping the stem cells' telomeres long? A healthy populace means the Social Security Trust fund need never be paid out and taxes could be collected indefinitely.

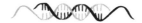

You Gotta Like Ike

Let us understand why the system is the way it is. For this, we need to remember what one of our finest presidents, Dwight D. Eisenhower, said in his Farewell Address to the Nation in 1961. For a career military man and reluctant politician, this would be the equivalent of calling his children and grandchildren to his bedside to impart his final blessing and some wisdom. Simply replace "arms" and "military" with "medical" and you will understand how I now view our system.

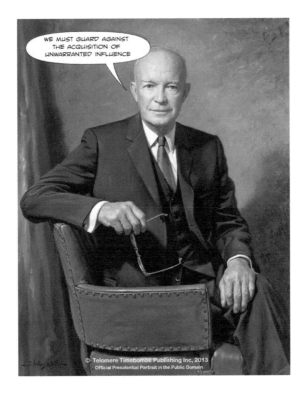

This conjunction of an immense military establishment and a large arms industry is new in the American experience. The total influence — economic, political, even spiritual — is felt in every city, every statehouse, every office of the federal government. We recognize the imperative need for this development. Yet we must not fail to comprehend its grave implications. Our toil, resources and livelihood are all involved; so is the very structure of our society. In the councils of government, we must guard against the acquisition of unwarranted influence, whether sought or unsought, by the military-industrial complex. The potential for the disastrous rise of misplaced power exists, and will persist.

— Dwight D. Eisenhower, 1961,
Farewell Address to the Nation

Disease Maintenance, Medical Research, and the How the Game is Played

In Washington DC, the most powerful lobbies are not patient advocacy groups or even physicians; they are the insurance companies and the drug companies. That should concern anyone worried about health care value because their motives are opposite those of the consumer, corporate health care buyer, and society in general.

The goal of an insurance company is to collect premiums and not pay out for health care. They refer to the money they expend on actual payments as the "medical loss ratio" so that if 80 cents of each dollar collected is spent paying for x-rays, medications, and doctor visits, then 20 cents are available for administration and profit.

The goal of a drug company is to develop proprietary new drugs that preclude lower profit margin sales of generic knockoffs for as many years as possible. It is during the exclusivity period that they can recoup the large research costs and feed profits. Even though existing drugs may have better safety and efficacy, the drug companies must push newer versions of perfectly fine older drugs so that they can satisfy shareholders.

There is no money in wellness. The big bucks are in the growth industry of illness or disease management. Massive donations flow in from walk-a-thons, collections, outreach, golf tournaments, etc. And to where do those dollars go? To academics who too may be working with drug companies to test exotic new molecules on patients who agree to experimental treatments because of blind faith or desperation. As I learned firsthand when my father was battling brain cancer, the more desperate you are, the less you can resist becoming fodder for fringe therapies that might spell your downfall.

Where is the money coming from to invest in health maintenance, healthy living and wellness?

The answer is, it comes from consumers because the FDA, the drug companies, insurance companies, and academic researchers can't monetize wheatgrass or meditation.

It is logical to say that if you can be diagnosed with a disease, then you can buy a pill. A new pill is more profitable than an old generic one although it is less time-tested and effective. Doctors are incentivized to push newer ones. If the new pill gives you a nasty side effect, then now the insurance company and you can purchase a second pill to manage the new complication. If the complication becomes a full-blown disease unto itself, guess what? More drugs! Once you get on the pharma train, there's no getting off until the last stop and that is a station you don't ever want to reach.

I am always proud of my patients who have resolved to stay off medications for as long as possible and who unabashedly challenge their doctors' efforts to add new meds. These people are consciously fighting the good fight of independent thinking and their bold actions are a daily inspiration to me.

The system would be more justifiable if academics' could coordinate their efforts in the most efficient and insightful ways possible. In point of fact, the most immediate of motivations are to publish papers that support their own ideas, that advance careers, create relationships with big pharmaceutical companies, and increase power and influence in academia and possibly within the secular world, like winning a Nobel Prize for instance.

Too often, the peer-reviewed publishing system is inefficient, competitive, and an exercise in game theory rather than a master-planned and coordinated campaign on a disease. Ike would have been displeased at the way medical research is conducted; it's like guerilla warfare waged in skirmishes. Like Hollywood studios working on similar scripts and racing through development, multiple labs compete to prove the same things or incrementally advance outmoded theories in deference to scientific orthodoxy.

Our representative government currently represents corporate interests all too well, in my opinion. The game played within the Washington Beltway (the circular highway surrounding the city) is one of swapping hats and stepping stones. I might start out life as low-paying government agency employee, then work for an insurance or drug company for a while, and then become a lobbyist to influence congressmen to legislate in my best interests. This is the ecosystem that Eisenhower was referring to and there is nothing inherently wrong with it. But the system does grant these "corporate citizens" incredibly loud voices when compared to individuals and that may not be in the best interests of the body politic when it comes to getting the best value for our health care dollars.

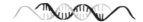

Prejudice Runs Deep

Research the discovery of TA-65 and look at the undeniable evidence that it enhances telomerase activity. It becomes hard to refute a potential mechanism for all the anecdotal improvements noted in the previous chapter and in my 45+ webinars on YouTube.

But the "too good to be true" doctrine trumps rational thought for most people. It seems that the degree of resistance towards the idea of safely restoring DNA and reversing aging is proportional to its desirability and years of education. And inversely proportional to the ability to exercise independent thought.

Every day someone tries to convince me that the sole reason telomerase-based anti-aging can't be true is because there have been so many shams that came before. That logic is extremely weak because it is easy-to-vary. If the "fool me once shame on you, but fool me twice, shame on me" doctrine were universal, then there could be no Jesus of Nazareth. There would be no 2004 Red Sox. There would be no happy second marriages.

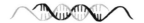

Spreading the Gospel before Nero Throws Another Garden Party

People ask me why I encourage so many doctors to compete with me in the selling of TA-65. As the first MD outside T.A. Sciences to be licensed to provide it, I have a huge head start so competition doesn't threaten me that much. But let's think about the market here. There are over 7 billion people who could benefit and they would want to take it forever!

Also, it is great karma to help patients become healthier, doctors become wealthier, and society to become wiser. But the most important reason I am scrambling to get the word out like Saint Paul on a whirlwind tour of the Mediterranean is the following:

What if there really was a safe way to prevent aging and stave off illness? Do you think that would be a welcome discovery for those who sell insurance and pills? I am racing to get the word out with this book and all the teaching I provide via videos and lectures because someday, someone will pick up the phone and ask to shut down the use of nutraceuticals in this manner. At that moment, I want so many of lobbyists, CEO's, and senators and their loved ones to be taking telomerase activators that they wouldn't dare make it unavailable or worse, illegal.

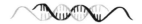

One Flew Over the Cuckoo's Nest

I mentioned that Soledad Mexia, the fifth oldest person in the world, was a patient and friend. She took TA-65 for three months and grew hundreds of jet black hairs. What I didn't mention is that she discontinued taking it, and why.

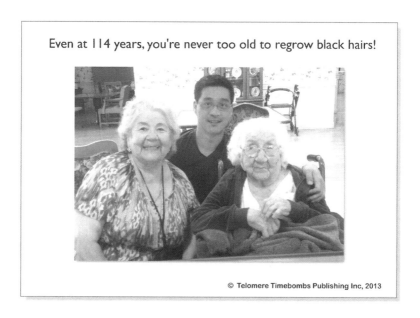

Even at 114 years, you're never too old to regrow black hairs!

© Telomere Timebombs Publishing Inc, 2013

Armida (80), Me (46) and Soledad (114)

Because her dreams became more vivid, she began talking in her sleep and disturbing her roommate. As a result, the facility decided to sedate her chemically.

Although safe and not a medicine, the nursing staff was not comfortable letting Soledad take a nutritional supplement so I spoke with the staff and called the attending physician. I explained the premise of telomerase activation medicine and sent him links to my website'but I never received any return calls.

When I spoke with her physician two years later he did remember me but didn't recall any instructions to forbid taking TA-65. Her daughter is 80-year-old Armida Galaz, and Armida told me that she was expressly forbidden from giving anything to her mother. She was worried that her mother would lose her spot at the nursing home if she disobeyed this prohibition on nutritional supplementation.

When I first gave it to Soledad in 2011, she healed some ulcers very quickly and her mood and mental status were good for her 112th birthday, singing and laughing with her family.

But when I revisited in Spring of 2013 to document the persistence of her black hairs, she looked tired and had a poorly healing infected skin abrasion on her only remaining leg. A similar problem led to an above-the-knee leg amputation a couple of years before I first met her.

We know what happens when people get old. When I first met her in 2011, she was the 18th oldest person in the world. In 2013, she was the 5th. That means thirteen people in their 110s died in the past two years.

It is sad that her family feels they are unable to explore this exciting option. Soledad is a treasure and she deserves to benefit from something that her family deems to be safe and beneficial and that is not a medication per se.

But like all but one of the inmates in the movie about an insane asylum breakout, *One Flew over the Cuckoo's Nest* (United Artists, 1975), everyone was there voluntarily and they had to play by the facility's rules to enjoy the protection of those walls. So in the end, we are all like inmates on Nurse Ratched's ward, taking our pills, watching the channel she wants to put on, and never questioning the authority of those we allow to control us.

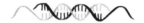

Coming Out of my Closet

They say people's number one fear is not death but public speaking. You will get no argument from me on that. I have to lecture in front of large audiences, host live webinars, and explain what I do to strangers but at my core, I am a very introverted and at times, cringe-worthy in my awkwardness.

During my years learning screenwriting as a craft, I watched a lot of movies and especially love the movies of the 1970's American New Wave like *Harold and Maude* (Paramount Pictures, 1971), *All that Jazz* (Columbia Pictures, 1979), and *Network* (MGM/United Artists, 1976). I suppose the reason for this book and my conscious choice to offer my introverted self into the public domain could be summarized by three catchphrases from those movies: "If you want to sing out, sing out," "It's showtime!," and because "I'm mad as hell and I'm not going to take this anymore!"

I'm sick and tired of patients running up against closed-minded doctors who bully them into giving up all hope of ever getting better before their inevitable and painful demise. The patients who come to me have already faced down and rejected institutionalized nihilism and could teach their doctors a lot about wellness. With the advent of telomerase activation medicine, I believe all the rules have changed and rather than walking obediently around the concrete structure of received medical wisdom, we can all take a cue from Roger Daltrey, himself a user of TA-65, and do what *The Who* did on their album cover for "Who's Next."

There is a war, my friends, and it is that war for the dignity of each human life that we will discuss in the next chapter. If what I am saying about telomerase activation medicine is true, I believe the war has already been won, even though the Medical-industrial complex might think of it as some rowdy kids throwing snowballs before the Battles of Lexington and Concord.

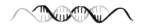

11

THE FUTURE

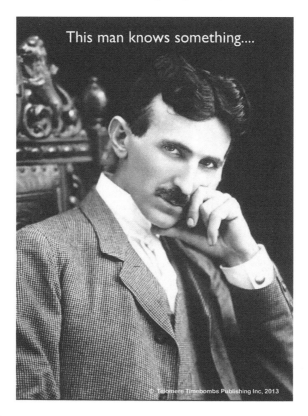

"The day science begins to study non-physical phenomena, it will make more progress in one decade than in all the previous centuries of its existence."

—Nikola Tesla

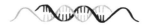

Now is the time to take a stand in your life and make a change. In this final chapter, I will discuss the new landscape of health and wellness, talk about holistic medicine, wax philosophically about the universe, and then give you some concrete steps to improve your understanding and your health now that you have taken the first step towards a life of true hope and abundance.

In the previous chapters, I have outlined our escape plan from the prison of hopelessness that we call modern medicine. You don't need to enter Andy Dufresne's tunnel, as in *Shawshank Redemption* (Castle Rock Entertainment, 1994) or jump on Chief's shoulders, as in *One Flew Over the Cuckoo's Nest* tonight and quite frankly, if you do nothing, I believe this revolution will catch up and overtake you soon enough.

The prison is in your mind and as Bob Marley told us "Emancipate yourself from mental slavery. None but ourselves can free our minds." Question authority. But question those who question authority too. Nobody has the monopoly on truth but in the end, I believe that my telomere/stem cell theory of aging and the hope it provides via telomerase activation is merely a statement of the obvious. The emperor has no new clothes, and the ideas in this book are not only "hard-to-vary," they are nearly IMPOSSIBLE-to-vary.

Jack Weinberg of the Congress on Racial Equality and Berkeley's Free Speech Protests once said "We have a saying in the movement that we don't trust anybody over 30." How old are you and your doctors now?

Even Ben Franklin may have to eat crow now. He quipped, "In this world nothing is certain but death and taxes." When I am asked, "Are there any negative effects of taking a TA?," I have inform them that yes, they may have to pay more taxes. Seriously, can you afford to live forever? What is the alternative?

And for those of you inclined to listen for the sound of other shoes dropping, here's your payoff from the *Twilight Zone* genre (television anthology, 1959-1964): the natural release from an unhappy marriage or the funding of an idle retirement are both at peril when the assumptions about your expiration date are altered in a fundamental way.

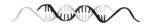

What is Holistic Medicine?

This very question belies its own ignorance. The better question is: "what ISN'T holistic medicine?" There is not a single malady that you can suffer that shouldn't be understood in terms of the whole individual. Genetic disorders of metabolism have inherent compensations that can mitigate them. Even poisoning is handled by the liver, intestines, and kidneys and regulated by the hormonal milieu. Cancer is the result of stress, poor telomere repair, and failed apoptotic systems. The list goes on and on.

There is a fitting quote that is often attributed to C.S. Lewis. It was first expressed in print by Scottish Minister George Macdonald:

"Never tell a child you have a soul. Teach him, you are a soul; you have a body."

—*The British Friend*, a British Quaker periodical,1892.

Truly, the consciousness of our body, mind, social identity, and environment all act in concert to determine the nature of our health and wellbeing just as it determines what diseases will afflict us in which order. And make no mistake, just as Irv Gordon would have collected nearly every type of automotive problem in 3 million road miles, you will get nearly all the diseases if you keep on surviving the ones that pop up due to shortening of the telomeres in your stem cells.

A holistic view suggests that "disease" is just that; the result of "dis-ease" in your life. It stands to reason that measures to restore ease, or balance and calm, will be healing in nature. There are so many people who claim to be healed of incurable afflictions by light, herbs, meditation, exercise, diet, and supplements and yet they are invariably painted with the "wacko" fringe label that short-circuits rational thought and replaces it with judgment.

The people who do their research and decide to try TA are a special breed that have the courage to think for themselves. Throughout the years, they have introduced me to areas of alternative medicine that I would have previously considered to be "out there" and incredible. But my promiscuous, "Why?" mind usually goes home and looks up what they are saying just to see if there is any kernel of truth or some new paradigm that I can pick up.

Some good examples of "fringe" medical thinking would be gluten and casein sensitivity, energy frequency Rife machines, and the dangers of genetically modified foods and radiofrequency waves.

But just because a David shouts down a Goliath, it doesn't make their conspiracy theory or pet remedy valid. By the same token, just because an authority labels something as non-scientific, doesn't mean it isn't worthy of study, like telomerase activation medicine.

My hope and expectation is that someday soon, the most reputable academic institutions with allied statisticians and clinical researchers will be collecting evidence with Level I randomized controlled trials involving TA for all the conditions that my Level III webinars describe. Based on my clinical experience, I am confident that even with small numbers of patients, measurable effects will be found in sleep, depression, exercise, nail growth and skin elasticity, sexual function, cold and flu frequency, and tolerance of chemotherapy.

In a blatant case of the cart being placed in front of Cinderella's mice, how many tens of millions of dollars were spent to prove it was healthy to ingest Resveratrol? That scientific debacle was just a proxy for red wine, which was a proxy for getting liquored up, in my jaundiced opinion.

Why not take a chance to disprove what I am suggesting or better yet, prove it true? The effects that I have seen are dramatic. I believe that in order to validate my telomerase activation hypothesis in many conditions, it would take only a year, perhaps only forty patients and a very modest amount of grant money to get your answers. But alas, these studies are impossible in the current climate. Why? Fear.

People are fear-based. These are the survival instincts, the lower chakras, the reptilian brains. What would be the fears associated of doing a randomized controlled trial to see if TA-65 does the things I have seen in my anecdotal cases?

Fear of hurting people or causing cancer, fear of being ridiculed and marginalized, fear of wanting to believe something so promising, fear of not being able to articulate why it is worth studying, fear of having to give up all the other paradigms of disease that they are clinging onto, and fear of losing money.

There is a school of thought that everything can be understood in terms of money. I don't subscribe to this idea but certainly, research departments are not going to get drug company funding to test telomerase activation if it is not a proprietary substance that can be exclusively patented. Remember that the main ingredient of TA-65 comes from a plant and is therefore an unregulated nutraceutical.

In the previous chapter we talked about the Medical-industrial complex and nothing better illustrates this than the drug approval process with the FDA (US Food and Drug Administration). It is supposed to protect the public interest by providing unbiased evaluation of the candidate drugs vying for approval.

But somehow the system was changed so that the drug companies pay the FDA. That seems like a good idea: if you are using government resources, then you should pay to keep the meter running. But paying to have your evaluation is like attending a school where the teachers are paid by the students. Can you say "conflict of interest?" I suppose it makes sense because soon enough the FDA regulators will be the ones working for the drug companies but perhaps there is a better way to safeguard the public interest?

Billy Crystal had a character on *Saturday Night Live* whose catchphrase was "It's better to look good than to feel good." Before I decided to focus on telomerase activation medicine, I was still offering lasers, botox, and injected fillers. Given the remarkable rejuvenation from taking TA-65, I invariably advised patients to spend the money on TA instead because it worked from the inside on the cellular level to improve the outward appearance with respect to wrinkles, hair and smiles.

It is interesting that the American consumer will spend billions on cosmetic procedures but will argue over a $15 copayment in the doctor's office. If people really understood how much TA could improve the quality of their life in a holistic way, I think they would make different choices on how their health and beauty money is allocated. If you ask me, it is better to feel good because the inner beauty generates outer appeal. But with TA, you don't have to choose because it both improves mood and makes you look better, in a safe and holistic way.

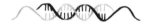

Life, the Universe and Everything

If you never stayed up late with intoxicated friends talking about what it all means or if you have never had goose bumps and experienced a sense that something just happened for a reason, you might want to skip this section.

In fact, I am cognizant that there are many personality types who may have often found themselves irked by my tone and my attempts at analogizing, irony or humor. To those people I wish to express my sincere gratitude for hanging in there. I hope it was worth it.

This is the part of the book that, depending on your philosophical and spiritual mileage, might seem like it doesn't belong. This book has been about science, aging, my crazy life, and a possible new paradigm for understanding and fixing the problem of getting sick and old. But as I have grown as a physician and a person, I have come to believe that some of the wacko theories that I used to mock may have some resonance after all.

I opened by telling you that I like to ask "Why?" Well, it turns out that when you try to explain why telomerase does what it does, or why the molecules can pull apart the chromosomes, there is no good explanation other than "consciousness."

A prominent expert in the field of consciousness, Dr. Stuart Hameroff of the University of Arizona, concluded that all of conscious life can be reduced to the microtubules. Microtubules organize into fibers that assemble then tether with great precision in order to allow for chromosome separation. They also give structure and motion to cells. And according to Hameroff, they allow for quantum level action on the neural plasticity of the mind. But why stop at that level? Why not discuss why the proteins that make up microtubules, tubulins, do what they do? How do they "know" what to do? Who "told them?"

You can reduce any argument to nonsense by going deeply enough. A famous thought experiment by Xeno (pronounced 'zeenoh') said if you travel half the distance to the ground for each unit of time, you would never reach the ground because there would always be another half to travel. But try jumping off a building and you might have a different opinion on that one.

If you expand upwards, many smug cosmologists and spiritual leaders say the universe is one panpsychic consciousness creating itself to experience itself? Why would an impersonal universe even care about what it manifests? Who is it trying to impress and who created it in the first place?

For the anthropomorphically-inclined monotheists, I was just participating in a thread on a social media site that asked: "if you could ask God anything, what would it be?" My comment was "Who created you? How do you know? Where will you go when you die? Don't you really pick sides (like the Israelites or the Crimson Tide) somewhat arbitrarily?" It all comes down to the scale in which you frame an argument, doesn't it?

One of the great stories of modern science is the attempt of our current secular religion, theoretical physics, to create a model that can "unify" the fields of gravity, electromagnetism and the strong and weak nuclear forces. Nikola Tesla, one of our greatest souls and minds, firing on all chakras, was quoted to open this chapter. Tesla was a gentleman with some serious "chops" when it came to physics, deep original thinking, and futurism and he was suggesting in that quote that we should study non-physical phenomena. There are many people working in fields of quantum energy, quantum consciousness, scalar waves and for the life of me, it all seems like nonsense to me.

And yet, it is undeniable that no philosophy, religion, theory or prejudice can explain why matter acts the way it does if it isn't just a little bit conscious, right? Hopefully, you are still a little bit conscious after having read the preceding paragraphs so I won't overstay my welcome into your attention span much longer.

In conclusion, I am left with only two truisms: everything is consciousness of a sort and the understanding of a system depends on framing and the scale of vision you are interested in. It would be absurd for a virus to contemplate black holes and it is probably equally absurd for you and me to ask why our universe was created.

Thankfully, there are clearer and more purposeful minds than my own who are busy elucidating the chemistry of cell function and genetic expression. And thankfully, there are deeper and wiser souls to express the connections and greater purpose of it all.

As I sit here typing this, hoping that my consciousness can resonate with yours, I only know two things: 1) I am grateful for my humble, chaotic, and possibly meaningless life; and 2) if I can aid you to increase your consciousness and bliss, it was well worth it.

A friend of mine once told me that her daily mantra for 49 minutes a day was to contemplate upon the following truths: we as people do not truly exist, that everything is happening automatically, that our thoughts are the result of an ancient mind that is seeing, hearing and doing and yet there is no seer, hearer or doer. I am still trying to understand what that means and why it makes me both happy and a bit sad. Maybe another few hundred years on my life expectancy will let me process it more fully.

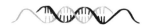

Back to Life, Back to Reality

This final section of this final chapter is all about concrete steps. I truly believe that negligible senescence is here, courtesy of scientifically-validated nutraceutical telomerase activation, and that this will change all the ground rules of the human condition. Can society afford to let everyone live forever? That was the question that led to the creation of my first screenplay and graphic novel, *Maximum Lifespan*.

Shameless plug alert! If you like serious science fiction, please **download *Maximum Lifespan* from iTunes as an app or buy a copy of my graphic novel** from my website, www.maximumlifespancomic.com. In that story, the wealthy elite are able to take telomerase activators and get caught growing lobotomized clones for replacement organs, prompting the angry masses to resent them and require physical separation outside the walls of the inner metropolis fortresses in every major city.

The billionaires of the 21st century foolishly tried to escape dying by having their heads cut off and frozen. Now in the 22nd century, they communicate with virtual reality interfaces and are conspiring to download their consciousness into unsuspecting bodies, just like the evil scientist father plans to do to his own son/clone.

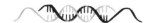

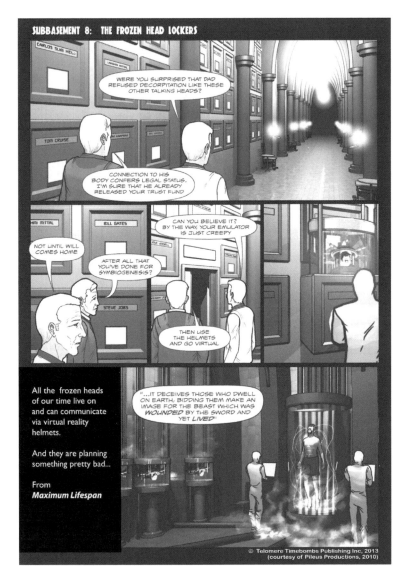

**What will become of today's über-wealthy
who buy into cryonics?**

Despite the scarcity of resources in my fictional world, I
believe that in the real world, life is abundant and on every level,

from the molecular to the cosmic, the universe is trying to help us rise and thrive.

In the near term, if TA does work the way I think it does, it will take some time to ramp up production of the Astragalus root and make it more affordable for everyone. Because of the current scarcity of the molecule in question, many people will likely die before they can benefit from this breakthrough discovery.

Let's talk about scarcity for a moment. There were plenty of times in the past few years that the scarcity of income and options might have caused me to give up on dreams of saving the world and even on myself. Circumstances and common sense might have frozen and constricted me into a lower consciousness of fear and scarcity.

So what was it that reminded me of the goodness and abundance of living? My patients. I would have the daily privilege of listening to my patients tell me how their lives had been transformed by telomerase activation. The truth is that where there is DNA repair, there is hope; where there is hope, there is life. So never ever give up hope on rescuing yourself and becoming the hero of your own journey.

They say when a person dies, it is like a whole library has burned to the ground. I wrote the Hypatia screenplay about the night they burned down the famed Library of Alexandria and martyred a great soul known as Hypatia. If you are interested in reading about the "tipping point" of Western history that plunged us into 1000 years of the Dark Ages, download my script at

www.pileusproductions.com/downloads/misc/NikesLastStand.pdf.

Shameless plug #2: if you would like to produce my screenplay or want to help me publish it as a novel, please contact me.

Proud plug: when a person deteriorates mentally and physically, it is like a nightly book burning at Nuremberg. To remedy this situation, I reserved the domain "Greatsouls.org" and my vision is to have an online platform like "Save the Children" but for grownups. They say that time is money, but now there will be a market to trade those commodities for the most "deserving" people we know.

The idea of Greatsouls.org would be to allow people to pitch their life stories so that others could make a personalized or anonymous donation to them through their webpage. Let's say someone across the world has a certain affinity for their classmates from their small high school, or they have always admired a type of unselfish person who pursued a career that they didn't because they were busy generating material wealth. Now they would be able to rebalance karma by exchanging money for health and vitality on behalf of others.

As the sponsored person's health and life begin to improve, video updates would be posted to their page and you can know that your tax-deductible donation is helping to keep a "Maha Atma" or great soul, alive and contributing to the world soul, such as it is.

I envision a vibrant community where people could socialize, reconnect, and celebrate with their many different social connections and show the world at large that aging and growing ill are truly a thing of the past.

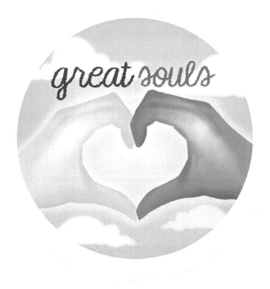

© Greatsouls.org 2013

Where there is love, there is hope

If, by the time you read this, Greatsouls.org is already up and running, please do go over and check it out to search for your ethnicity, your childhood neighborhood, your classmates or old friends, and whatever types of people you find noble and worthy of extra innings in this magnificent game of life.

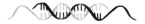

Live Long and Prosper

In order to live your longest and healthiest life, you must think for yourself. Cancel your subscription to a reality that says you are doomed to age and become ill. And question any authority that is giving you easy-to-vary theories that ignore the obvious importance of telomere damage.

Most importantly, trust but verify. Use your internet search engine to look up my videos, TA-65, telomeres, telomerase, and try to find anyone credibly alleging that this is a scam. Also go to PubMed and type telomere and any disease you wish. There will be MANY articles and nearly all of them will suggest a link to shortening telomeres.

Go to my website, www.RechargeBiomedical.com and watch my videos on a variety of topics. They are easy to understand, original, and I believe highly entertaining. With over 120,000 views on YouTube in two and a half years, it's not as viral as "Gangnam Style" or "Charley Bit my Finger" but it is not a bad effort for a middle-aged one-man show from Orange County. My channel on YouTube is "*drpark65.*"

And if and when you are ready, call my office and set up a phone consultation. Try to come in and have your biomarkers measured to establish a baseline age of your organs and possibly do a measurement of your LTL as well.

Then, try a proven, not a phony, telomerase activator to see if what I'm saying is true. The proof of the pudding is in the eating and in most cases, you will feel the improvements in sleep and mood immediately.

Let us remember the immortal words of one mortal poet, Dylan Thomas (from "Do not go gentle into that good night"):

> *"Do not go gentle into that good night,*
> *Old age should burn and rave at close of day;*
> *Rage, rage against the dying of the light."*

Your books are not ready to burn and the library should stand a while longer. We need you so don't give up hope.

Whether you live thirty more years or three hundred, I hope that you will please cherish every moment of your abundant life and be grateful, gracious and loving towards yourself and others.

We close with the words of someone who figured it all out without the benefit of few hundred antediluvian years:

> *"You can search throughout the entire universe for someone who is more deserving of your love and affection than you are yourself, and that person is not to be found anywhere. You yourself, as much as anybody in the entire universe deserve your love and affection."*
>
> — Syd ("don't call me the Buddha") Gautama

Thank you for taking the time to read my book. It was an honor and a blessing to be able to share what I believe is the most important information that you need right now in order to live your best and healthiest life. I hope our paths will cross someday and that when we meet, in the same way we now joke about dialing a phone or putting out the bottles for the milkman, we will laugh about the days when we actually concerned ourselves with shopping for funeral plots instead of stylish new bathing suits.

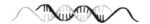

EPILOGUE

I am told that the countless eerie synchronicities that occurred while creating this book are signs that the universe is pleased that it was created.

As for forward progress, I realized that I was probably on the right path when I encountered Schopenhauer's second stage of ridicule. After I requested a blurb about my review copy of "Telomere Timebombs," a prominent figure in the anti-aging field replied:

> *"It is full to the rafters of the sort of egregious*
> *oversimplifications and prematurely confident conclusions*
> *that have blighted the public face of gerontology for*
> *decades"*

Perhaps men of letters are quick to condemn because they harbor a thermodynamic-like belief about truth: "I can't be right unless someone else is wrong."

Admittedly, there is much that I don't know about stem cells, telomerase activity and its regulation, and epigenetics but with each year, greater minds than mine bring us closer to understanding thanks to their deductive (top-down) scientific methods. Perhaps that is why the scientist who disliked this book was so offended. In his worldview, science must be specialized, incremental, and never overreach.

In my defense, I believe that good clinical medicine, like the creation of a new "telomerase activation medicine paradigm," requires inductive (bottom-up) reasoning. Thoughtful observations from anecdotes coalesce into patterns that we recognize, which then lead to working hypotheses. Where is the experimental validation for what I've written? That is not my expertise but I honor those who will follow and do the groundwork required to get everyone on board with this new paradigm for health and wellness.

I believe that when we can understand the behavior of cells more like the behavior of social insects, then we will be even closer to wisdom. Instead of the anthropomorphizing rampant in this book, we just need to "walk a mile" in the shoes of our cells. Oops, I guess I did it again...

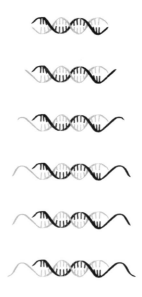

-Dr. Ed Park, August 11th, 2013